Books by Melissa C. Bernstein, OT, FAOTA

The Power of 5 Test Kitchen Cookbook—Caregiver Edition

The Power of 5 Test Kitchen Cookbook—Full Edition (Coming Soon!)

The Power of 5: A Journal for Health, Longevity and Wellness, Co-authored with David Bernstein, MD

Books by David Bernstein, MD, FACP

I've Got Some Good News and Some Bad News: YOU'RE OLD—Tales of a Geriatrician

Notes of Living Longer

Senior Driving Dilemmas: Life Saving Strategies

The Power of 5: The Ultimate Formula for Longevity and Remaining Youthful

The Power of 5: A Journal for Health, Longevity and Wellness, Co-authored with Melissa Bernstein

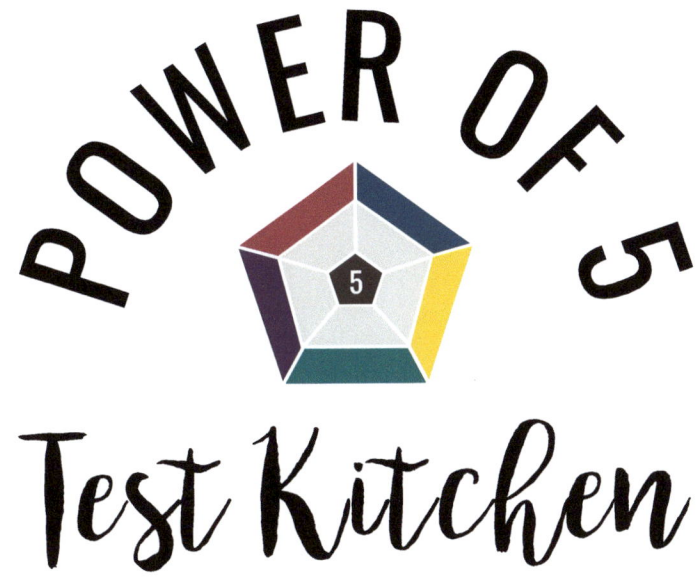

CAREGIVER EDITION

Melissa C. Bernstein, OT, FAOTA

Copyright ©2021 by Melissa C. Bernstein, OT, FAOTA

All rights reserved. No part of this publication may be reproduced or transmitted in any form or by any means, electronic or mechanical, including photocopying and recording or by any information storage and retrieval systems now know or to be invented, without permission from the publisher except for brief passages in connection with a review written for inclusion in a magazine, newspaper or broadcast.

Published in the United States by Dynamic Learning

Paperback ISBN: 978-0-9962322-8-9
E-book ISBN: 978-0-9962322-9-6

Books are available in quantity for promotional or premium branded corporate use.
For more information on discounts, terms and media requests contact:

Dynamic Learning
Media Department
314 Shore Dr. E. Oldsmar, Florida 34677-3916
813.922.2876

Visit us at: **Powerof5TestKitchen.com**

All Photos were taken by Melissa Bernstein

Dedication

To all the selfless caregivers who dedicate their lives to caring for those with neurodegenerative disease or other debilitating illnesses.

May the *Power of 5 Test Kitchen Cookbook* bring you joy and fun the kitchen as you cook with the individuals in your care.

Melissa

Table of Contents

Foreword 9-10

To Get Us Started 11
    The Basics of Collaboration Between Caregiver and Individual in the Kitchen 12
    Compassionate Cueing Techniques 13
    Types of Assistance Levels During Cooking 13

Let's Get Cooking

Breakfast Bites 15
    Protein Pancakes 16
    Fresh Vegetables on Avocado Toast 17
    Just Eggs Veggie Omelet 18
    Fresh Mixed Berries 19

Healthful Beverages 21
    Delicious Healthy Smoothies with Options 22
    Superfood Kale Smoothie 23
    Virgin Margaritas 24

Appetizers/Starters 25
    Mock Chicken Liver (not liver) 26
    Roasted Polenta topped with Mushrooms & Scallions 27
    Bruschetta 28

Salads for Any Meal 29
    Chickpea Salad 30
    Quinoa Salad 31
    Cool Health Salad 32
    Mexican Chopped Salad 33

Soup Warms Your Being 35
    A Heart-Healthy Veggie Soup 36-37
    Healthy Lentil Super Soup 38-39
    Gazpacho Soup 40

Sauces & Dippers 41
Traditional Mexican Guacamole 42
Pico de Gallo/Salsa 43
Easy Hummus 44

Main Dishes That Can Be Sides 45
Cheese and Vegetable Quesadillas 46-47
Stir Fry Veggies with Grilled Tofu 48-49
Light Eggplant Parmesan 50-51
Sheet Pan Fajitas 52-53
BBQ Grilled Kebabs 54-55

Sides That Can Be Main Dishes 57
Sheet Pan Roasted Green Beans and Baby Potatoes 58
Elote – A Mexican Street Corn Dish 59
Quinoa with Roasted Vegetables 60
Roasted Italian Zucchini 61

Snacks Can Be Healthy 63
Heart-Healthy Snacks 64
Dr. B's Brain Health Trail Mix 65
Grilled Fruit – Easy to Prepare and Delicious 66

Yes ... Healthy Desserts Please! 67
Non-Dairy Frozen Fruits Ice 68
Oatmeal Fruit Bake 69
Berries Yogurt Parfait with Dark Chocolate Drizzle 70
Homemade Applesauce with Strawberries 71

Closing Tastes: Thoughts from Melissa 73

Resources 75
Healthy Eating on a Daily Basis 75-77
Abilities Skills Inventory 78-79
Sample Adaptive Utensils and Equipment 80-82

With Gratitude 83

Contact Information 84

Foreword

I developed *The Power of 5 Ultimate Formula* for a broad and inclusive audience. As a geriatrician, I've observed first-hand the formulas that healthy seniors I've cared for have followed, enabling them to age gracefully. Throughout my career I've immersed myself in medical and scientific literature to understand the most common illnesses facing industrialized countries and the behaviors that are most likely to have a favorable impact on younger adults as they age. My major focus has been to improve and lengthen the human health-span, or the part of a person's life during which they are generally in good health. Even though I regularly treat illnesses in our aging population, it's best to start creating good habits early in life to achieve the optimal health-span.

My 40 years spent as a practicing physician has given me the unique perspective to track health trends that I highly recommended to a younger population. I've taken to heart much of what I have learned and adjusted my own lifestyle; incorporating those healthy components of *The Power of 5* that were missing in my life. My personal goal is to enhance my own health-span and share my knowledge about this subject with the world. All of my own nutritional choices are presented in *The Power of 5* and are incorporated in the concepts of *The Test Kitchen*. Motivation is key; therefore, setting personal goals and tracking them will enhance the likelihood for success. I have set personal goals that include traveling, spending time with family and educating the world. *The Power of 5 Ultimate Formula* emphasizes getting more Sweat, Sleep and Socialization and reducing Sweets and Stress.

I encourage readers of this cookbook to use *The Power of 5 Ultimate Formula for Longevity and Remaining Youthful* as a reference and motivation to make healthy lifestyle choices. What we eat is an incredibly important component of *The Power of 5 Formula*, and this book provides an excellent starting point. This cookbook is unique because it provides delicious recipes for a senior population that are simple, with a few ingredients. Steps for preparation are easy and designed to encourage participation from individuals with neurodegenerative diseases. The idea is to promote a collaborative activity that is both meaningful and fun. The selection of ingredients, which include reduced sugars and carbohydrates, will reduce the buildup of undesirable metabolic waste products in the brain and thus lessens the burden of the disease process.

Melissa Bernstein has an extensive background as an occupational therapist. She is engaged in many facets in her field and also has the rare distinction of being dually certified as a therapist entrepreneur and a chef. She has been cooking healthy meals throughout her adult life. After lending her cooking expertise as a natural collaborator to *The Power of 5* (she is also my wife); she was an obvious choice to develop recipes to support health and longevity in an aging population. Melissa founded *The Power of 5 Test Kitchen*, where she blogs about healthy food and posts her multifaceted recipes. After an avalanche of favorable responses to her food blogs and recipes, she embarked on publishing this cookbook. Melissa's work in *The Power of 5 Test Kitchen* is a shining example of how we can incorporate healthy eating into new and improving lifestyle choices. This cookbook provides a guide to eating clean during meals; focusing on our recommended mix of 30% proteins (fish, tofu, eggs or egg substitutes), 20% fruit (fresh not dried), 20% whole grains carbohydrates (grains, quinoa, beans or legumes) and 30% fats (avocado/olive oils).

Melissa and I have curated recipes in this cookbook that meet my criteria as healthy choices (according to a physician.) Melissa promotes and presents a Mediterranean, vegan and plant-based lifestyle proven most effective to prevent illness, reduce disease burden and has a favorable impact on the aging brain. She offers "Melissa's Modifications" for those who want options based on their own dietary preferences. For example, avoidance of certain allergens, gluten-free, dairy free, and consideration to add meat, fish, or poultry to satisfy individual tastes and meet the special needs of older adults. Older adults often have diminished sense of taste and smell which can affect palatability. Food consistencies might be a major concern if a swallowing disorder exists. Adults with neurodegenerative disease have even more specialized needs. This group of patients has a tendency to crave sweets. Melissa limits carbohydrates and sweets in most of the Test Kitchen recipes, but they are even more restricted for this patient group. The brains of older adults, especially those with dementia, do much better with diets higher in fat and lower in carbs, sweets and sugar. Melissa and I have provided recipes that might appear to be higher in fat and lower in sugar for this very reason.

The Power of 5 Test Kitchen Cookbook—Caregiver Edition provides tested, delicious recipes that are easy to make and guaranteed to satisfy anyone to whom you will serve. This cookbook offers the caregiver valuable resources to use when cooking with individuals who have neurodegenerative disorders to promote purposeful engagement.

David Bernstein, MD

To Get Us Started

Welcome Caregivers!

Persons who have neurodegenerative disease such as dementia, Alzheimer's disease, Parkinson's disease and other conditions may experience loss of memory as well as motor impairments.

In addition, concentration, feelings of anxiety, loneliness, and fear are just a few of the non-motor symptoms that may afflict an individual at different times and at different stages of the disease process. Guided activities of engagement such as cooking are safe and beneficial to the individual and the caregiver.

I am so excited to bring you the first of its kind published cookbook, offering a delicious means to incorporating purposeful engagement and socialization through food and cooking. I have specifically designed this cookbook for caregivers who are caring for an individual with neurodegenerative disease.

Eating for your health is very important for everyone and especially for anyone fighting a disease and especially when cooking for individuals with neurodegenerative disease … **Research has shown that a diet** high in protein, low in carbohydrates and little or no sugar provides the most favorable outcomes.

My profession, occupational therapy, speaks volumes to how to promote engagement and participation in meaningful activities. The essence of occupational therapy, what we do as healthcare professionals is to help people across their lifespan to engage and participate in things they need **or want to do through therapeutic use of everyday Activities of Daily Living (ADLs)**—dressing, bathing, personal hygiene, functional mobility, cooking, and eating/feeding—**the "occupation" of living.**

Instrumental ADLs (IADLs) supports daily life within the home and the community that often requires more complex interactions than those used in basic ADLs—two examples that speak to the purpose of this cookbook is **Care of Others** and **Meal Preparation.** Both of these higher-level ADLs encourage participation and engagement.

Food is powerful … it comforts.
It is a modulator of the mind-body connection.
It brings people together.
It stimulates our senses: taste, smell, vision, and hearing.
Food facilitates past reminiscences and is a powerful way of bringing memories back to life.
Using music during activities can instantaneously bring us back to those special recipes our family cooked, triggering the memories of what, when and where we experienced that meal.

Therefore, using food and cooking and eating with individuals with neurodegenerative disease is beneficial at many levels.

The Basics of Collaboration Between Caregiver and Individual in the Kitchen

Here are some general pre-cooking "MUST DOs" before we get started ...
- Be sure bathroom needs are met.
- Always wash hands before food prep.
- You and your cooking partner may want to wear disposable latex or allergen-free gloves during prep and handling of food.
- Hair should be pulled back if necessary.
- Always use compassionate cueing techniques with your cooking partner; the cornerstones are respect and safety.
- Use an apron if available to protect clothing during the cooking process.

My #1 rule in cooking is ... always be prepared!
While cooking always use a "Person-Centered Approach": especially for caregivers doing a cooking activity with individuals with neurodegenerative disease.

Additional Rules For Cooking in the Kitchen ...
2) **Perform the Abilities Inventory Form (see references section).** Before a cooking activity, explore likes/dislikes. Keep cooking activity appropriate for the level of the individual.
3) **Break the recipe down into bite-sized steps.**
4) **Patiently explain/discuss with the individual** what foods will be used to prepare the recipe and how you're going to take one step at a time.
5) **Pre-prepare if necessary,** keeping time in mind so as not to overwhelm or frustrate with a recipe with too many parts to complete. This is very necessary for individuals who may have shortened attention spans or who demonstrate apprehension or even fear.
6) **Encourage involvement in all steps** of the preparation. Even if they are unable to assist, engagement at any level is meaningful.
7) **Stay focused on the individual's** physical and mental engagement throughout the purposeful activity.
8) **Remember oven/kitchen utensil safety.** The caregiver may have to handle some parts of the cooking activity based on skill level of the individual with neurodegenerative disease.
9) **Caregivers must keep an eye out for fatigue/attention** and adjust as you feel necessary to maintain the engagement of the individual to the activity.
10) **Consider and plan the ambiance of the setting and conversations starters** to enhance the cooking and dining experience, making it enjoyable, memorable and fun! Once the food is completed, you will be ready to enjoy the foods of your labor. And lastly, but extremely important ...
11) **Take time to talk** about the making of the recipe. What were the parts they liked the best?
    Reinforce reminiscing and engagement and, most importantly, **dining with dignity** as you plan your next cooking experience!

Compassionate Cueing Techniques

Compassionate cueing techniques, as I call them, are core principals for caregivers to keep in the forefront when working with those with neurodegenerative disease.

- Respectful at all times when communicating during a task or activity.
- Accept the level of where they are and work from there.
- Gentle guidance and suggestions will help to ease successful completion of steps of a task.
- Never force or disregard feelings if they resistant, retreat and try a different approach.
- Remember – safety first, with kitchen appliances, utensils, and positioning while cooking.

Types of Assistance Levels During Cooking

While cooking, you may have to provide some verbal or physical guidance throughout a cooking activity for engagement. Here are some general assistance levels that may come into use during cooking.

- *Supervision Only* – no physical assistance, independently completes the activity
- *Verbal Cueing* – needs verbal instructions of the steps to complete the activity
- *Minimal Assist* – minimal hands-on assistance or guidance with verbal instruction to complete the activity
- *Moderate Assist* – requires some verbal instruction and physical assistance to complete the activity
- *Maximum Assist* – cannot complete task without maximum verbal instruction and maximum physical assistance throughout the activity

Let's Get Cooking

Breakfast Bites

- Protein Pancakes
- Fresh Vegetables on Avocado Toast
- Just Eggs Veggie Omelet
- Fresh Mixed Berries

POWER OF 5
Test Kitchen

Protein Pancakes

A healthy and delicious breakfast packed with 46.4g of protein, low in carbohydrates and very flavorful. Inspired by Training4Fitness, adapted in the **Power of 5 Test Kitchen**. Other alternatives to make your pancakes non-dairy, you can find under my Melissa's Modifications section ... Enjoy!

PREP TIME	COOK TIME	PASSIVE TIME	SERVES
10 minutes	15 minutes	0 minutes	2

INGREDIENTS

- 1/2 cup protein powder (I replace with peanut butter protein powder for added flavor)
- 1/2 cup almond flour
- 1/2 tsp sea salt
- 10 drops stevia (liquid) or half banana (I prefer the banana)
- 4 large eggs (see notes for non-egg option)
- 1 cup cottage cheese, low-fat variety or homemade dairy-free (see notes)
- 1 Tbsp coconut oil

INSTRUCTIONS

1. Combine the protein powder, almond flour, baking soda and salt in a medium bowl. Mix until fully combined.
2. In a food processor combine the stevia, eggs, cottage cheese and milk. Add the dry ingredients and pulse to combine.
3. Heat a pancake griddle over medium heat. Grease with the coconut oil, cook the batter by ¼ cup scoops until bubbles form, then flip and cook the other side until golden.
4. Serve with olive oil or grass-fed butter.

MELISSA'S MODIFICATIONS

I love these pancakes, I use peanut butter protein powder for added flavor rather than plain protein powder. Additional alterations that can be made:

Vegan non-dairy options: For egg replacement, try using "chia egg" which is made from taking 1 Tbsp of chia seeds + 1 Tbsp of lukewarm water, mixed and allow to gel.

For cottage cheese: It is very easy to make your own non-dairy cottage cheese using silken tofu and spices blended until everything is smooth. Here is what you will need:

- 1 300g block soft or silken tofu (about 1 1/3 cups)
- 1 Tbsp nutritional yeast
- 1 tsp apple cider vinegar
- 1 tsp lemon juice
- 1/2 tsp salt
- 1/2 of a 420g block firm tofu (210g or about 1 1/2 cups), crumbled

Instructions:

Add the soft or silken tofu to a blender along with the nutritional yeast, apple cider vinegar, lemon juice, and salt. Mix until everything is completely smooth, stopping to scrape the sides as needed. Pour the soft tofu mixture into a medium bowl. Crumble the firm tofu into the silken tofu mixture. Mix to combine.

NUTRITIONAL VALUE | 1 serving
Calories 488, Fat 24.4g, Carbohydrate 382g, Protein 48.4g

Fresh Vegetables on Avocado Toast

Avocado toast with sautéed veggies is my most favorite meal – breakfast, lunch or dinner! Quick, easy and delicious!

PREP TIME
15 minutes

COOK TIME
10 minutes

PASSIVE TIME
0 minutes

SERVES
1

INGREDIENTS
- 1/2 cup spinach, chopped
- 1/4 cup broccoli florets
- 4 large mushrooms, sliced
- 1/2 medium tomato, chopped
- 1-2 slices Dave's Killer Bread® 21 Grain and Seeds is my favorite, but any whole grain bread or rye toast works just as well!
- 1/2 avocado, sliced
- 1 slice onion, chopped
- 1/2 green pepper, chopped
- 1 Tbsp olive oil (Alternatively, you can sauté with water or Bragg Liquid Aminos.)
- Everything But The Bagel Seasoning, to taste

INSTRUCTIONS
1. Take all veggies except for the avocado and sauté lightly on high heat with olive oil (water or Bragg Liquid Aminos).
2. Toast the Dave's Killer Bread® or whole-grain bread of your choice.
3. Spread the avocado on the toast, put the sautéed vegetables on top and enjoy!
4. Sprinkle with Everything But The Bagel Seasoning for added flavor. Can you tell I love this seasoning? My favorite!

MELISSA'S MODIFICATIONS
Simple ingredients, easy to prepare, and delicious! Feel free to add other veggies of your choice in the sauté.

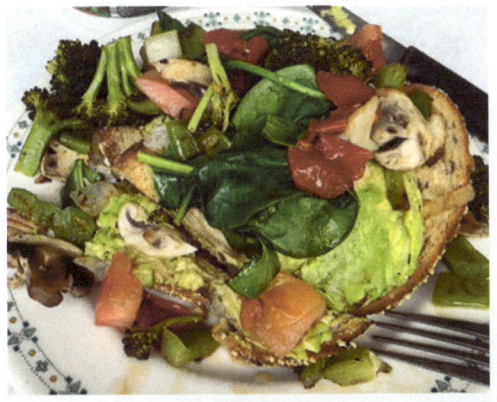

NUTRITIONAL VALUE | 1 serving
Calories 232, Carbs 22g (Fiber 8.4g), Protein 6g

Just Eggs Veggie Omelet

My favorite way to prepare Just Eggs is with sautéed onions & mushrooms with avocados, on toasted Dave's Killer Bread® 21 Whole Grains and Seeds.

PREP TIME	COOK TIME	PASSIVE TIME	SERVES
15 minutes	10 minutes	0 minutes	2

INGREDIENTS

- 12 Tbsp Just Eggs (6 Tbsp Just Eggs = 2 regular eggs)
- 1 small onion, diced
- 1 cup mushrooms, chopped
- 1 whole avocado, sliced (try California or Florida avocados – they are large, less dense and have less calories)
- Cheese, optional (cheese of your choice)
- 1–2 Tbsp organic vegetable broth as needed so onions/mushrooms do not stick to pan

INSTRUCTIONS

1. On the stove top, in a large saucepan, medium heat, sauté onions until brown, adding a little veggie broth so it does not stick to the pan.
2. Add mushrooms and continue to sauté until done.
3. Lower the heat and add the Just Eggs over the onion and mushroom sauté.
4. Let sit for 3-5 minutes, moving the pan side to side to move liquid to sides. Use spatula to lift up sides to assist in cooking.
5. When Just Eggs is nearly cooked, with spatula, carefully release one side, then the other to be able to fold over.
6. If you want cheese, you can sprinkle inside before you fold over or on top once folded.
7. Place sliced avocados on the top.

MELISSA'S MODIFICATIONS

The Just Eggs also can be scrambled with a variety of other sautéed vegetables, add cheeses of your choice as well. I have used Just Eggs in quiche, and other baked goods requiring eggs. I even used to make matzoh balls when making matzoh ball soup, and they held their form in the soup.

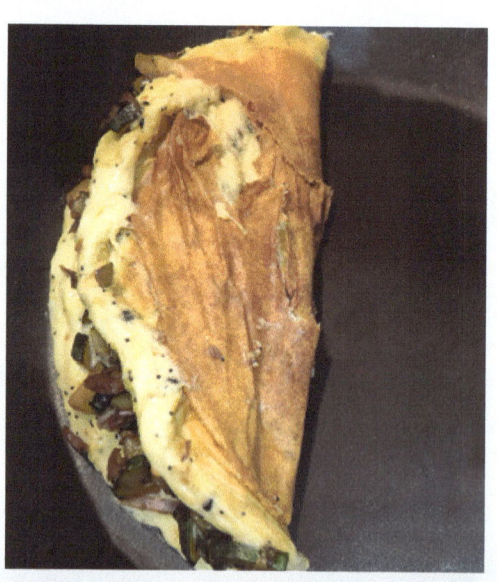

NUTRITIONAL VALUE | 1 serving based on 2 eggs (6 Tbsp Just Eggs) 321 Calories; 24g Fat; 329mg Sodium; 7.3g Carbs; 7.6g Fiber; 2.7g Sugar (natural); 13g Protein. (Avocado included) One slice of Dave's Killer Bread - Thin sliced - 60 Calories; 1g Fat; 9g Carbs; 3g Fiber; 3g Protein.

Fresh Mixed Berries

Mixed berries make a light breakfast bite, filled with vitamins, minerals, antioxidants, fiber and natural sugars. For added protein add a dollop (about 2oz) of plain yogurt or low-fat cottage cheese.

PREP TIME	COOK TIME	PASSIVE TIME	SERVES
10 minutes	0 minutes	0 minutes	4

INGREDIENTS
- 1 cup blueberries
- 1 cup strawberries, hulled and sliced
- 1 cup blackberries
- 1 cup raspberries
- 1 tsp lemon juice, fresh
- 8 oz yogurt, plain or vanilla, optional
- 8 oz cottage cheese, low-fat, optional
- 1 Tbsp hemp heart seeds, chia seeds, pumpkin or sunflower seeds, if desired

INSTRUCTIONS
1. Wash berries and pat dry
2. Hull the Strawberries and slice as desired
3. Mix together in a bowl and toss lightly
4. Serve 1/4 of the berries in a bowl, top with 2 oz of yogurt or low-fat cottage cheese.
5. Sprinkle with seeds of your choice for added protein, if desired.

MELISSA'S MODIFICATIONS
Fresh berries in the morning are a great start of your day. Easy to prepare and with added yogurt and nuts give you added vitamins, protein (especially the hemp hearts, which add fiber and antioxidants. The yogurt and cottage cheese can be non-dairy if you are vegan or don't eat dairy.

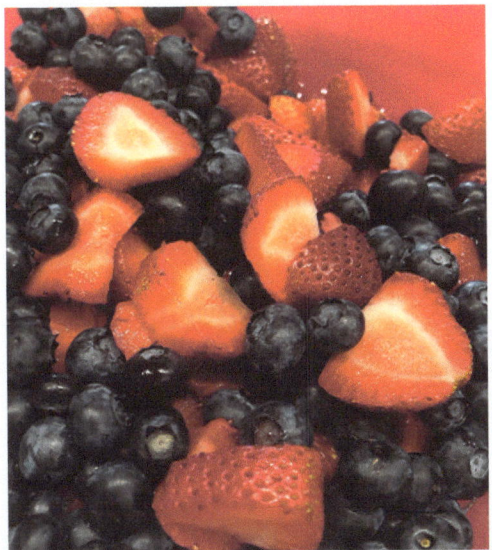

NUTRITIONAL VALUE | 1 cup serving
122 Calories; 0 Cholesterol; 1.3mg Sodium; 17.7g Carbs- 6g Fiber, 10.4g Sugar; 4g Protein.

Healthful Beverages

- Delicious Healthy Smoothies with Options
- Superfood Kale Smoothie
- Virgin Margaritas

POWER OF 5
Test Kitchen

Delicious Healthy Smoothies with Options

Here are the basics of a super healthy and delicious smoothie!
Each ingredient has options based on your tastes.

PREP TIME
15 minutes

COOK TIME
0 minutes

PASSIVE TIME
0 minutes

SERVES
1

INGREDIENTS

- 1/2 cup unsweetened almond, cashew, rice, soy, hemp, or low-fat milk, or coconut water
- 1 cup frozen sliced banana
- 1/2 cup frozen fruit; blueberries, cherries, strawberries, pineapple, mango, apples, raspberries, blackberries, grapes
- 1/3 cup protein powder (your choice); pea protein powder if you are vegan; other proteins such as whey if you eat dairy
- 1 cup greens, kale or baby spinach
- 1 Tbsp chia seeds, flax seeds or nut butters (a bonus) for healthy fats and a little more protein

INSTRUCTIONS

1. Throw all items in the blender, blend until the desired consistency. Add more water if it gets too thick.
2. Pour in a mason jar (my favorites storage containers for smoothies and soups) cover and go!

MELISSA'S MODIFICATIONS

LIQUID: Choose unsweetened non-dairy milk of your choice. Juice is too high in sugar to use (even if they are 100% juice).

FROZEN BANANA: Naturally sweet, always rich, and add creaminess.

FROZEN FRUIT: Using frozen fruits make a frosty smoothie. Use ice if you want your smoothie very icy! I buy organic frozen berries for ease and freshness.

PROTEIN: A must for staying-power! Protein will slow digestion of carbs which will keep you fuller longer.

GREENS: Using a cup of kale or baby spinach helps to add veggies to your day without dominating the smoothie.

ADDED POWER: Throw in some chia, flax or hemp seeds for a boost of fiber and added nutrition (Omega 3s) or nut butters (almond, peanut or cashew) for added protein.

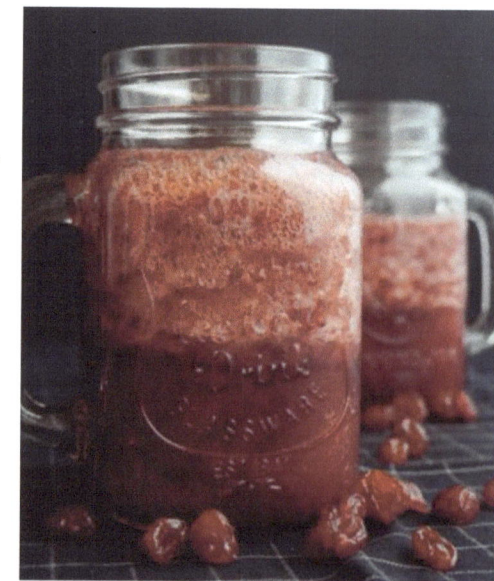

NUTRITIONAL VALUE | 1 serving
Calories 232, Carbs 22g(Fiber 8.4g), Protein 6g

Superfood Kale Smoothie

Kale, spinach or other deep green vegetables eaten in any form adds so many beneficial vitamins, minerals and antioxidants to enhance ones overall health. Add kale, spinach or other dark green vegetables to your diet.

PREP TIME	COOK TIME	PASSIVE TIME	SERVES
5 minutes	0 minutes	0 minutes	1

INGREDIENTS
- 1 handful kale or spinach
- 1 tsp ginger, 1/4 inch piece of peeled ginger
- 1 cup pineapple cut, fresh or frozen
- 1 cup coconut water any flavor, I use pineapple flavor
- 1 tsp spirulina powder, optional (I put extra in mine, noted by the dark green color!)
- 1 tsp wheatgrass powder, optional
- Slivered nuts, optional
- 1 scoop protein powder, optional for added protein

INSTRUCTIONS
1. Add all ingredients in your blender and blend until smooth.
2. If it is too thick, you can always add more water or ice.
3. For an added boost of fiber add Flax or Hemp seeds.
4. Once prepared, top with gogi berries, flakes of coconut or slivered almonds (or cashews), pomegranate seeds, or even berries of your choice.

MELISSA'S MODIFICATIONS
Smoothies are a great way to add nutrition to your diet, replenish after a workout or as a meal replacement. Add protein powder like Orgain brand to increase the protein, and decrease the fruit to decrease carbs and fats.

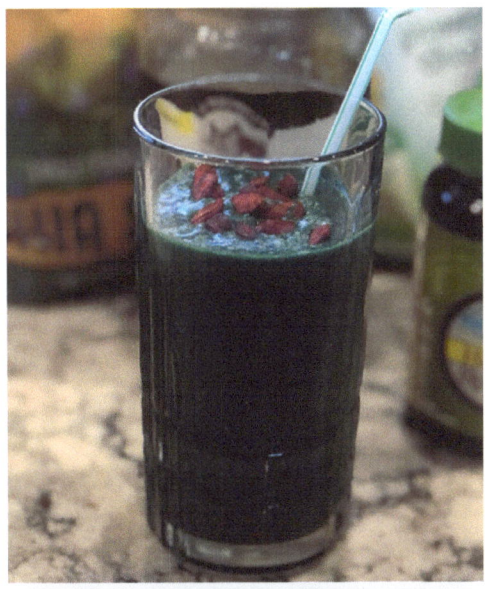

NUTRITIONAL VALUE | As prepared 337 Calories; 9.4g Fat; 26g Carbs; 18g Fiber; 30g Protein. If the calories are too high, adjust the ingredients to decrease carbs and increase protein.

Virgin Margaritas

Margaritas are a fresh citrus drink delicious for Cinco de Mayo celebration, virgin or with a little Jose Cuervo Tequila ... refreshing at any time.

PREP TIME	COOK TIME	PASSIVE TIME	SERVES
20 minutes	0 minutes	0 minutes	4

INGREDIENTS

- 1/2 cup lime juice
- 1/2 cup lemon juice
- 1/4 cup superfine sugar, or more to taste
- Crushed ice
- Club soda
- 4 lime wedges, optional
- 1 Tbsp kosher salt, optional

INSTRUCTIONS

1. **Make the lemon-lime mixture.**
   You have two options here: on the rocks, or frozen. The rocks version is the easiest and least time-consuming way to make a virgin margarita.
   Simply combine the lime juice, lemon juice, and sugar (or substitute) in a small pitcher, stirring until the sugar has dissolved.
   For Margaritaville-style frozen drinks, blend the lime juice, lemon juice and sugar with 4 cups of ice in a high-powered blender. Blend until the mixture is nice and slushy.
2. **Prepare the glasses**
   For a true margarita experience, you'll want to prepare a salted glass. This step is optional, of course, but it does make the glasses look fancy.
   Start by swiping one of the lime wedges around the rim of the glass. Then, pour some coarse salt onto a small plate and dip the edge of the glass into the salt, rolling it around until the edge is coated.

MELISSA'S MODIFICATIONS

To reduce sugar, substitute with 6–8 drops of Stevia Clear. The natural sweetener has zero calories and offers plenty of sweetness to balance the tartness of the lemons and limes.

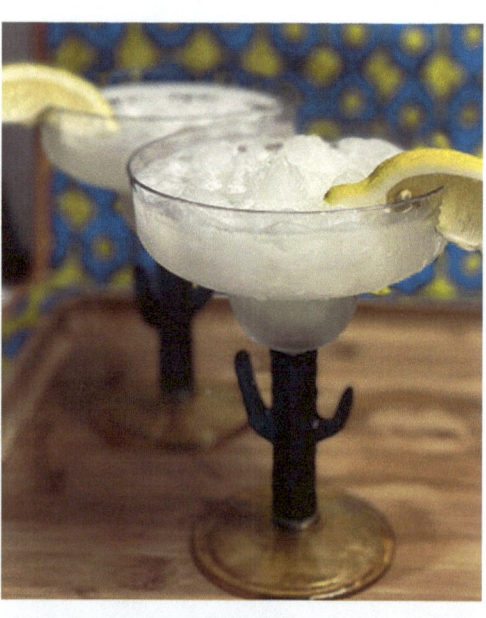

NUTRITIONAL VALUE | 1 serving The virgin version is barely any calories, especially using Stevia Clear. Add 4oz of 90-proof tequila, 90 proof and this adds 300 Calories and 28g of Carbohydrates! Stick with the virgin version ... better for you!

Appetizers/Starters

- Mock Chicken Liver (not liver)
- Roasted Polenta topped with Mushrooms & Scallions
- Bruschetta

POWER OF 5
Test Kitchen

Mock Chicken Liver (not liver)

A flavorful appetizer as a start of any meal. I usually prepare this when my kids are home for the holidays. Easy to make and the recipe goes a long way.

PREP TIME
20 minutes

COOK TIME
5 minutes

PASSIVE TIME
0 minutes

SERVES
8

INGREDIENTS
- 1 large can cooked peas
- 1 Tbsp oil to sauté the onions
- 2 large onions, chopped
- 1/2 cup walnuts, chopped
- 3 hard-boiled eggs, use 1 egg yoke and whites from the eggs; omit if you are vegan
- Salt & pepper to taste

INSTRUCTIONS
1. Sauté onions in the small amount of oil until brown and crisp.
2. In food processor, chop peas, walnuts and eggs. Do not puree – leave mixture somewhat grainy.
3. Add onions with a bit of the oil.
4. Blend a few seconds until the mixture is well blended but you can still see a few flecks of egg white (no worries about this if you omitted the eggs) and brown onions.

MELISSA'S MODIFICATIONS
This is a delicious recipe that can be served with any veggies as a dip, Mary's Gone Crackers (my favorite), matzo, or any cracker for that matter. I have even used it as a spread on a sandwich with lettuce and tomato. Give that a try with the leftovers (if there are any) the next day on two slices of Dave's Killer Bread®, 21 Whole Grains with Seeds Thin Sliced. Very yummy!

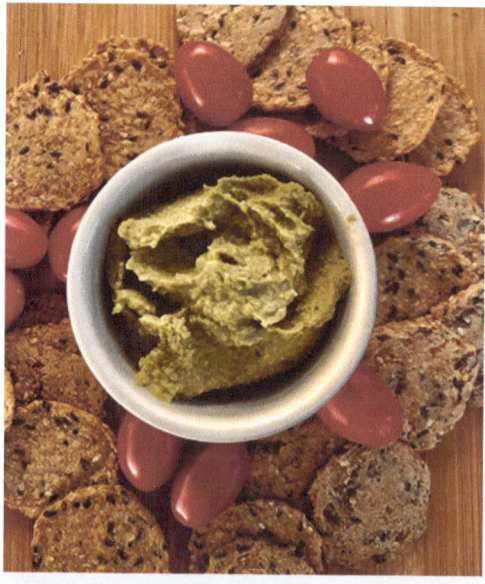

NUTRITIONAL VALUE | 1 serving (full recipe with eggs) 122 Calories; 7.5g Fat; 23.2mg Cholesterol; 178.3mg Sodium; 5g Carbs; 2g Fiber; 4.6g Protein. **No Eggs -** 104 Calories; 6g Fat; 0 Cholesterol; 140.5mg Sodium; 5g Carbs; 2g Fiber; 2.5g Protein

Roasted Polenta topped with Mushrooms & Scallions

Polenta is a versatile foundation upon which you can layer many delicious ingredients to put together a great appetizer or main course.

PREP TIME
15 minutes

COOK TIME
10 minutes

PASSIVE TIME
0 minutes

SERVES
4

INGREDIENTS
- 2 18.1 oz rolls polenta, cut into 1/2" slices
- 1–2 lbs gourmet mushrooms: an assortment oyster, cremini & shiitake mushrooms, cut into thick slices
- 2 scallions, thinly sliced
- Extra-virgin olive oil
- 1/2 cups chopped parsley
- 4 oz Fontina cheese or similar
- 1/2 teaspoon crushed red pepper
- 1/4 cup sherry vinegar
- Kosher salt & pepper
- 1/2 cups tomato sauce, I like the organic brands with added basil if I am using store-bought sauce

INSTRUCTIONS
1. Preheat oven to 450°F.
2. Slice the polenta into 1/2-inch slices or 1/2-inch thick rounds.
3. Brush both sides lightly with olive oil and place on a rimmed baking sheet covered with parchment paper. Roast until golden brown and warmed through, about 25 minutes.
4. Meanwhile, in a large skillet, heat the oil over medium heat and add mushrooms. Stir often until tender and slightly browned, about 12 minutes.
5. Add cut shallots, vinegar, salt, and red pepper. Sauté for about 5 minutes. Stir in parsley.
6. Place a teaspoon of tomato sauce on each slice of roasted polenta.
7. Divide mushroom mixture and spoon over the tomato sauce.
8. Top with cheese and continue to roast in the oven until cheese is melted, about 5 minutes.

MELISSA'S MODIFICATIONS
I love the ease of using polenta as a base for this delicious mushroom and scallion mixture. You can make the mushroom mixture a day or so ahead if you want to save time preparing. Store the mixture in an airtight container in the fridge. There are so many other topping options. Use any sautéed vegetables or pasta sauce with a slice of sausage and cheese on top. I have also made a "meatless" lasagna layering polenta instead of using lasagna noodles.

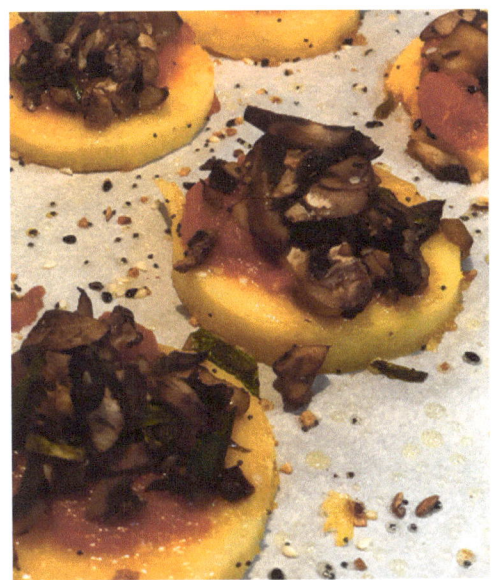

NUTRITIONAL VALUE | 1 serving 2 pieces of polenta - 132 Calories; .7g Fat; 0 Cholesterol; 47g Carbs; 3g Fiber; 11g Protein.
Add cheese on top - add 2 tsp Fontina cheese on top of one serving - 18 Calories; 1.4g Fat; 5.2mg Cholesterol; 36mg Sodium; .1g Carbs; 1.2g Protein.

Bruschetta

There's nothing like a delicious tomato bruschetta on a piece of crusty rustic bread! It's so very good as a starter.

PREP TIME 15 minutes **COOK TIME** 0 minutes **PASSIVE TIME** 0 minutes **SERVES** 4

INGREDIENTS
- 1 loaf crusty or rustic bread, cut into thick slices
- 1 - 2 cloves garlic, make into a garlic paste
- 3 - 4 Tbsp extra-virgin olive oil
- 3 large tomatoes, ripe and juicy
- 1 small bunch fresh basil, tear into pieces
- Part-skim mozzarella cheese or Parmesan cheese, optional
- 1 pinch salt as needed

INSTRUCTIONS
1. Dice the tomatoes and put in a bowl. Add the torn basil leaves.
2. Chop garlic. Sprinkle a pinch of salt on top, then smear the salt into the garlic with the flat side of a knife until a paste is created and the juices have released from the garlic.
3. Add garlic paste to the tomato mixture.
4. Add pinch of salt and pepper along with 3-4 Tbsp of olive oil. Mix together well. Let the mixture marry for 5 minutes or so.
5. Slice the bread, and grill on both sides until both sides are crusty but soft enough in the middle.
6. Grate fresh garlic on the bread.
7. Scoop tomato mixture onto the bread. Garnish with fresh basil as desired.

MELISSA'S MODIFICATIONS
This is a simple and easy recipe to prepare and serve. As a modification to this recipe, I have added fresh mozzarella or Parmesan on the top, then broiled for a few minutes to melt the cheese before serving. If you do not eat dairy, use Violife plant-based cheeses. They are great alternatives. You can also make a cashew-nut-based ricotta cheese, which you can find on the Power of 5 Test Kitchen website.

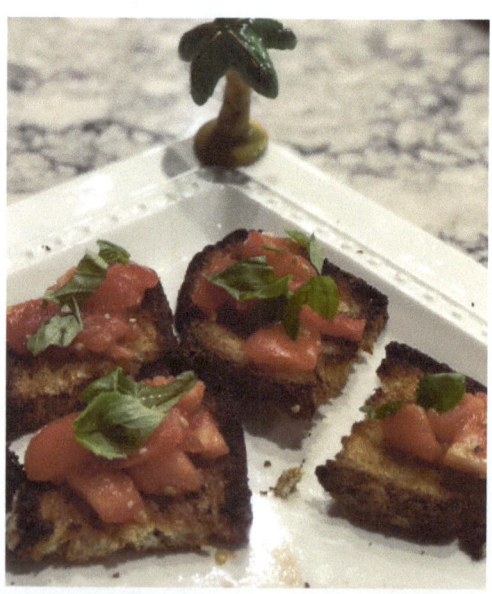

NUTRITIONAL VALUE | 1 serving 123 Calories; 9g Fat; 3g Carbs; 1g Fiber; .8g Protein
With Added Violife plant-based cheese: 137 Calories; 10.2g Fat; Sodium 36.4mg; 3.9g Carbs; 1g Fiber; .8g Protein

Salads for Any Meal

- Chickpea Salad
- Quinoa Salad
- Cool Health Salad
- Mexican Chopped Salad

POWER OF 5
Test Kitchen

Chickpea Salad

Chickpea salad is a quick and easy way to enjoy a heart-healthy lunch filled with fiber and important nutrients. So many ways to enjoy!

PREP TIME
10 minutes

COOK TIME
0 minutes

PASSIVE TIME
0 minutes

SERVES
3

INGREDIENTS
- 1 can organic garbanzo beans/chickpeas
- 2 stalks celery, chopped finely
- 1 medium carrot or shredded carrots, about 1/4 cup
- 1 small onion, chopped finely
- 1 tsp spicy brown mustard or to taste
- 2 Tbsp avocado mayonnaise, regular or vegan
- Salt and pepper

INSTRUCTIONS
1. Put the well-rinsed chickpeas and chopped vegetables into a food processor. Pulse a few times to combine, but do not over blend.
2. If you don't have a food processor, you can use a mixer, Magic Bullet blender, or mortar and pestle, or you can chop all veggies and chickpeas together until they are combined.

MUSTARD/MAYONNAISE DRESSING
3. In a separate mixing bowl, mix mustard, mayonnaise and seasonings. Add more of one condiment than the other based on your preference. I love mustard, so my chickpea salad is heavy on the spicy brown stuff!
4. Add dressing to the chickpea and veggie mixture and stir until well-blended. Serve on a bed of lettuce with added veggies or half of a pitted avocado!

MELISSA'S MODIFICATIONS
If you do not like chickpeas, you can replace them with baked tofu. Butter beans also make a smooth and flavorful replacement. There would be no need to put these through the food processor as they are very soft and can be hand mixed.

Another option to try is jackfruit, which I have talked a lot about in my food blogs ... this also does well as a replacement and is packed full of nutrition.

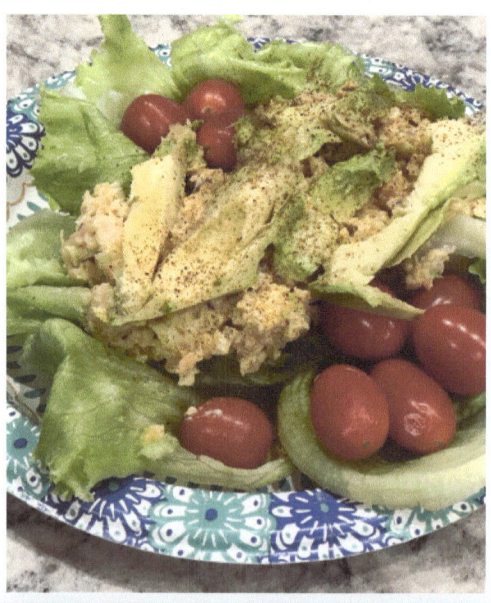

NUTRITIONAL VALUE | 1 serving
9.2g Fat; 286mg Sodium; 20g Carbs; 8.8g Fiber; 7.8g Protein

Quinoa Salad

A refreshing salad loaded with protein, vitamins and minerals.

PREP TIME	COOK TIME	PASSIVE TIME	SERVES
10 minutes	15 minutes	0 minutes	4-6

INGREDIENTS

- 1 cup dry organic quinoa; red, multi blend or regular – your choice
- 1 cup of vegetable broth
- 1 cup water
- 3/4 cup cherry tomatoes, sliced in two
- 1/2 cup red onion, chopped
- 3/4 cup shredded carrots, for ease I buy the already shredded ones
- 1 avocado, peeled and diced
- 2 Tbsp balsamic vinegar

INSTRUCTIONS

1. Cook the quinoa according to package with the vegetable broth and water for 15 minutes until all quinoa is absorbed. Let cool.
2. In a large glass bowl, add cooled quinoa.
3. Cut up cherry tomatoes, red onion, avocado.
4. Add all cut up veggies and shredded carrots to the bowl of quinoa.
5. Pour the balsamic vinegar over the mixture and gently mix all together.
6. Serve over a bed of lettuce.

MELISSA'S MODIFICATIONS

Quinoa is a low-glycemic superfood that is full of protein and fiber and is a great source of antioxidants and minerals such as iron, magnesium, folate, zinc and copper.

It is so versatile it can be eaten hot or cold like this dish. Add veggies, additional proteins such as tofu, chicken, or fish.

You can make a batch on Sunday and eat in a variety of ways during the week.

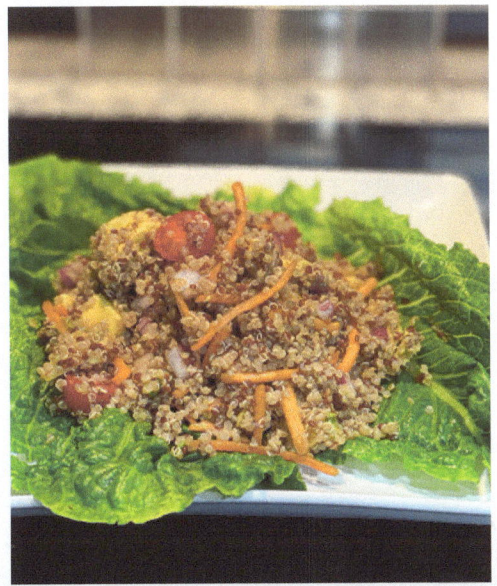

NUTRITIONAL VALUE | 1 serving
194 Calories; 8.4 Fat; 0mg Cholesterol; 54.4mg Sodium; 27g carbs; 7.4g Fiber; 5g Protein.

Cool Health Salad

A refreshingly cool health salad is the perfect summer recipe. This salad has fresh, crisp, succulent vegetables. When blended together, they provide a flavorful and hydrating meal.

PREP TIME	COOK TIME	PASSIVE TIME	SERVES
20 minutes	0 minutes	0 minutes	4

INGREDIENTS
- 1 medium cucumber, diced
- 1 can black beans, I use low sodium
- 1 1/4 cups corn, roasted or canned
- 1/2 cup purple onion, diced
- 1 cup cherry tomatoes, sliced in half
- 1/2 cup cilantro, chopped (I am not a fan of cilantro, so I left it out of my salad)
- 1 lime or lemon, if desired
- 1–2 avocados, diced
- Salt and pepper to taste
- Pinch chili power, optional, to add a zip, as desired
- Everything But The Bagel Seasoning (One of my favorites! This added flavor!)

INSTRUCTIONS
1. Place the diced cucumber, black beans, corn, cherry tomatoes, chopped onions, and cilantro in a bowl.
2. Squeeze fresh juice from the lime onto the salad.
3. Mix well together.
4. Add chopped, diced avocado. Season with salt, pepper and other suggested seasonings.

MELISSA'S MODIFICATIONS
You can add other veggies to this salad, such as sweet peppers, artichokes, and/or hearts of palm (which we love) for an added boost. Many other veggies pair nicely with this salad.

For our favorite light vinaigrette – use olive oil, lemon juice, and spices of your choice. A splash of balsamic or apple cider vinegar can also be added to taste.

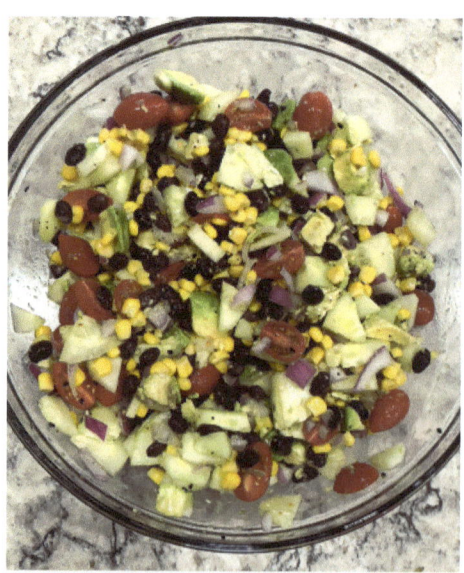

NUTRITIONAL VALUE | 1 serving
Calories 274; Fat 11g; Fiber 9g; Carbs 37g; Cholesterol 0; Sodium 24mg; Potassium 935mg; Sugar 6g; Protein 9g.

Mexican Chopped Salad

A protein-packed, flavorful salad. A meal in itself!

PREP TIME
45 minutes

COOK TIME
10 minutes

PASSIVE TIME
0 minutes

SERVES
4-6

INGREDIENTS
- 2 fresh ears corn, roasted on the grill or steamed, cut off the cob
- 2 hearts romaine finely shredded, about 5 cups
- 1/2 14 oz can black beans drained & rinsed
- 1/2 cup cherry tomatoes, halved
- 4 scallions, white and green parts only, thinly sliced
- 1 ripe avocado, diced
- 1/4 cup cilantro, roughly chopped

Green Goddess Dressing
- 1/4 cup sheep or goat milk yogurt or Vegenaise to make it vegan
- 1/4 cups cilantro
- 2 scallions, white and green parts only, chopped
- 1/2 green jalapeños roughly chopped (or use more or less to taste)
- 1/4 cup lime juice, freshly squeezed
- 1/2 cup extra-virgin olive oil
- 1 Tbsp raw honey

INSTRUCTIONS
DRESSING
1. Combine all ingredients in a powerful blender and pulse until completely smooth.

SALAD
2. Steam or grill the corn until cooked. When cool enough to handle, slice kernels off the cob.
3. Place the shredded lettuce in a large bowl and add all other prepared ingredients. Toss with 1/2 of the dressing or to taste.

MELISSA'S MODIFICATIONS
This recipe is packed with protein and can be 100% whole food plant-based by using Vegenaise (low-fat) in the dressing instead of mayonnaise. If you do not avoid dairy, then no alterations are necessary. Use dressing sparingly as it is high in calories (and is very rich, so lightly dress the salad and you'll have plenty of flavor), or use a low-fat/low-cal green goddess dressing.
If you feel you need added protein, then add grilled organic chicken or grilled tofu.

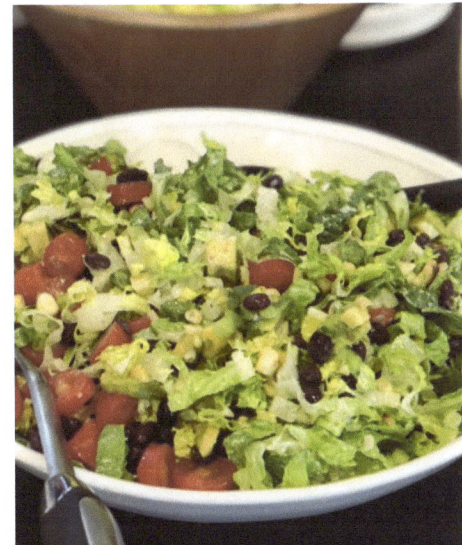

NUTRITIONAL VALUE | 1 serving *Salad:* Calories 163, Fat 8.3g, Sodium 120g, Carbs 15.2g, Fiber 7g, Protein 5.2g
Dressing as recipe directed: 1.5 tablespoons ~ Calories 121, Sodium 136.3g, Fat 12.3g, Carbs 3g, Protein .1g

Soup Warms Your Being

- A Heart-Healthy Veggie Soup
- Healthy Lentil Super Soup
- Gazpacho Soup

POWER OF 5
Test Kitchen

A Heart-Healthy Veggie Soup

A one-pot concept is so versatile. This can be made on Sunday, making many meals for the week or to freeze. Heart-healthy recipes full of fresh vegetables, whole grains, legumes or other proteins ... what could be better? I am providing lots of options to create your healthy soup to your taste. Print out the ingredient list and choose your items to include prior to making it. You can make a very light soup with just one grain, no potatoes, or make it more hearty with multiple beans. Items marked ** are choices based on your taste as you build your heart-healthy soup!

PREP TIME	COOK TIME	PASSIVE TIME	SERVES
30 minutes	2 hours	0 minutes	8

INGREDIENTS

- 4 – 6 cups, choose your base of soup broth **I begin all my soups with a vegetable broth base. You can use chicken or beef broth too.
- 4 medium potatoes, chopped **I prefer sweet potatoes as they sweeten the soup. Red or gold potatoes also work well.
- 2 15 oz cans cannellini beans **Optional, instead of potatoes or quinoa. Other options are kidney, garbanzo or pinto beans.
- 2 medium – large onions, chopped
- 8 yellow squash and/or green zucchini, sliced; add broccoli, cauliflower, green beans if you wish
- 4 whole carrots, chopped
- 1 cup quinoa or black rice, uncooked
- 1 15 oz can diced or crushed tomatoes, undrained
- 1 cups kale and/or spinach
- 10 – 16 oz added protein of your choice **Chicken, fish, sausage or plant-based meats. If not precooked, be sure to do that before you add to soup.
- 1 can tomato paste
- 4 cloves garlic minced or 4 – 6 tsp of already minced garlic, based on taste
- Ground black pepper to taste
- Smoked paprika to taste, optional
- Water as needed
- 1 – 2 Tbsp curry, tumeric, cumin, depending on your taste; adding one of these spices can add flavor and health benefits
- 2 Tbsp extra-virgin olive oil as needed
- 1 – 2 Tbsp Bragg Liquid Aminos or low sodium soy sauce (a healthy replacement for salt)
- 1 – 2 Tbsp Bragg Nutritional Yeast Seasoning, adds great flavor to food; salt-free, sugar-free, gluten-free, vegetarian and kosher!

A Heart-Healthy Veggie Soup

INSTRUCTIONS
1. All soups start with prep of your veggies. Making a big pot of heart-healthy soup is so easy. Choose your soup base, then add in veggies and proteins prior to cooking. I've provided options to make a delicious soup no matter what ingredients you choose to add.
2. Slice, chop your veggies of choice.
3. Saute onions, carrots and potatoes with vegetable broth or olive oil for a few minutes to get the cooking process started.
4. If you add quinoa or rice, you can prepare beforehand, following the package directions or, my preferred method, just add additional water to the soup and cook along with the other ingredients.
5. If you add organic beans to the soup, be sure to rinse beans prior to adding to soup.
6. In a large stock pot, add soup broth, spices, all sautéed and chopped vegetables, beans, and grain of choice.
7. Add pre-cooked meat the last 15 minutes of soup cooking time. If not pre-cooked, such as most plant-based products are, cook them first. Either sauté with seasoning or buy already cooked.

MELISSA'S MODIFICATIONS
I make delicious soups several times a week as a main meal or side dish to accompany our dinner. I hope you will enjoy tapping into your creativity by choosing your ingredients to build a delicious soup this weekend!

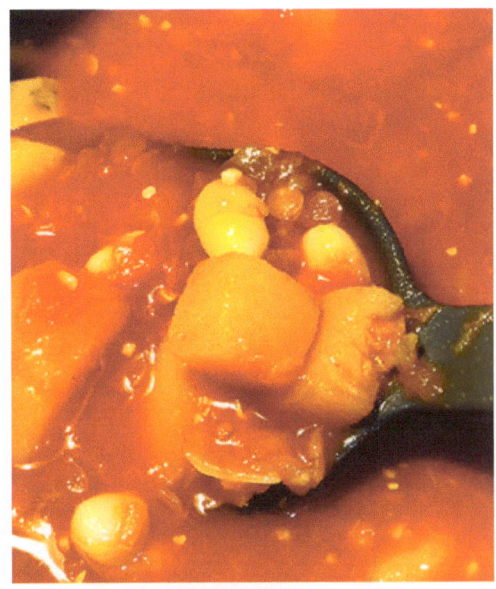
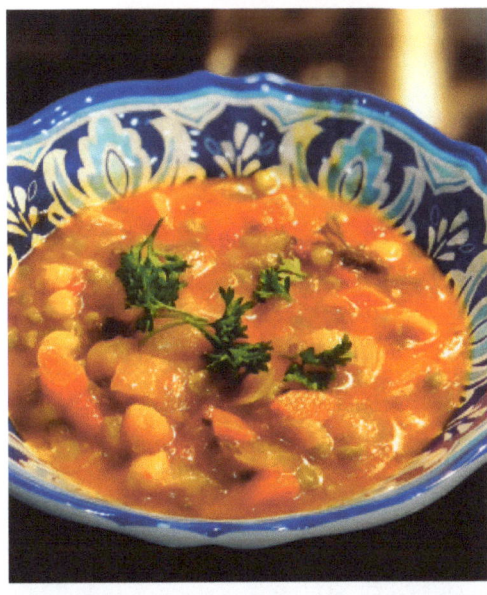

NUTRITIONAL VALUE | 1 serving
224 Calories (no meat);1.6g Fat; 0mg Cholesterol; 104mg Sodium; 50.8 Carbs-9.6g Fiber, 9.9g Sugars; 10.4g Protein.

Healthy Lentil Super Soup

Lentils are a healthy superfood … an anti-inflammatory food rich in protein, fiber, iron, B6, folate and antioxidants. Lentils are edible seeds from the legume family. They do not require soaking before using, and they cook to a creamy soup that is very easy to prepare.

PREP TIME	COOK TIME	PASSIVE TIME	SERVES
15 minutes	30 minutes	0 minutes	6

INGREDIENTS

- 1 Tbsp extra virgin olive oil
- 1 medium sweet yellow onion, about 1 cup chopped
- 2 carrots, peeled and chopped
- 2 celery stalks, chopped
- 3 garlic cloves, pressed or minced
- 1 tsp ground cumin
- 1 tsp curry powder
- 1/2 tsp dried thyme
- 1 large can (28 oz) diced tomatoes, lightly drained
- 1 cup dry red or green lentils, picked over and rinsed
- 4 cups vegetable broth
- 1 cup water, may need more depending on thickness preferred
- 1 tsp salt, more to taste
- 1/4 tsp of cayenne pepper or red pepper flakes, more can be added if you want more heat
- Freshly ground black pepper, to taste
- 1 cup chopped fresh kale, tough ribs removed, or spinach
- 1 to 2 Tbsp lemon juice (1/2 to 1 medium lemon), to taste

INSTRUCTIONS

1. Warm the olive oil in a large Dutch oven or pot over medium heat.
2. Once the oil is shimmering, add the chopped onion and carrot and cook, stirring often, until the onion has softened and is turning translucent, about 5 minutes.
3. Add the garlic, cumin, curry powder and thyme. Cook until fragrant while stirring constantly, about 30 seconds. Pour in the drained diced tomatoes and cook for a few more minutes, stirring often, in order to marry their flavors.
4. Pour in the lentils, broth and the water. Add 1 tsp salt and a pinch of red pepper flakes. Season generously with freshly ground black pepper.
5. Raise heat and bring the mixture to a boil, then partially cover the pot and reduce the heat to maintain a gentle simmer. Cook for 25 to 30 minutes, or until the lentils are tender but still hold their shape.
6. Transfer 2 cups of the soup to a blender. Securely fasten the lid, protect your hand from steam with a tea towel placed over the lid, and purée the soup until smooth. Pour the puréed soup back into the pot. (I use an immersion blender to blend a portion of the soup.)
7. Add the chopped greens and cook for 5 more minutes, or until the greens have softened.

Healthy Lentil Super Soup

8. Remove the pot from the heat and stir in 1 Tbsp of lemon juice.
9. Season to taste.
10. Serve while hot. Leftovers will keep well for about 4 days in the refrigerator, or can be frozen for several months (just defrost before serving).

MELISSA'S MODIFICATIONS

There are many varieties and colors of lentils; brown, red, yellow, green which are the most popular. Yellow and red lentils are split and cook quickly. Lentils can be made to add protein to a delicious salad, used as a base of a spread or dip, uses for this versatile. They are high in fiber and support a healthy bowl and growth of healthy gut bacteria.

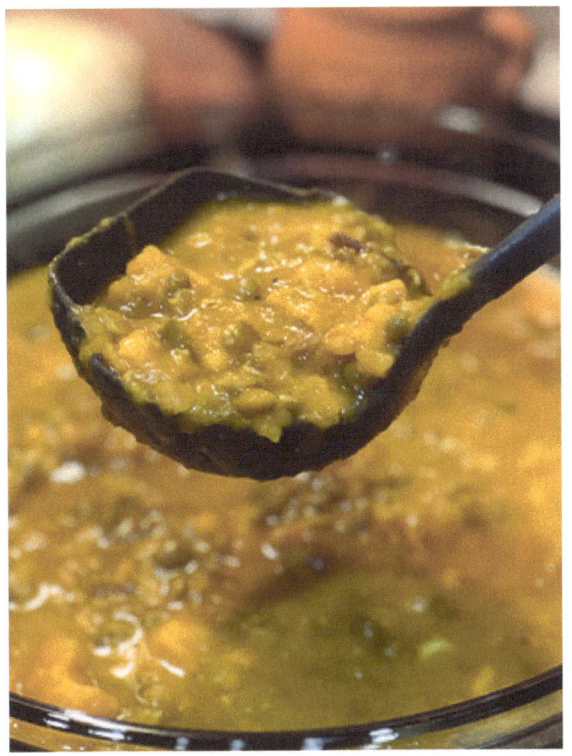

NUTRITIONAL VALUE | 1 serving
366 Calories; 15.5g Fat; 0mg Cholesterol; 47.8g Carbs – 11g Fibers, 10.8g Sugars; 14.5g Protein.

Gazpacho Soup

An easy-to-make cold soup that also may be served hot!

PREP TIME
20 minutes

COOK TIME
30 minutes

PASSIVE TIME
0 minutes

SERVES
8

INGREDIENTS

- 2 lbs ripe red tomatoes, cored and roughly cut into chunks
- 1 medium cubanelle pepper or another long, light green pepper, cored seeded and roughly cut into chunks
- 1 medium cucumber, peeled and roughly cut into chunks
- 1 small onion (white or red), peeled and roughly cut into chunks
- 1 clove garlic
- 2 tsp sherry vinegar, more to taste
- Salt
- 1/2 cup extra-virgin olive oil, more to taste plus more for drizzling
- 6 or more drops Tabasco sauce, to taste
- 1 tsp Worcestershire sauce, omit if you follow a vegan, vegetarian or gluten-free diet

INSTRUCTIONS

1. Combine tomatoes, pepper, cucumber, onion and garlic in a the blender. Blend at high speed until very smooth (about 2 minutes).
2. With blender running, add vinegar, salt, Tabasco, Worcestershire sauce. Slowly drizzle in the olive oil. The mixture will turn dark pink or bright orange as it becomes smooth.
3. Strain the mixture through a strainer pushing the liquid through with a spatula or back or ladle. Discard the solids.
4. Transfer to a large glass pitcher and chill until very cold. At least six hours or overnight.
5. Before serving, add additional seasoning if desired. If soup is very thick, add a little bit of ice water.

MELISSA'S MODIFICATIONS

This very low-cal soup filled with vitamins and antioxidants is a summer favorite. I often like to keep my Gazpacho chunky, omitting putting through the blender. If you prefer this texture, chop all the vegetable in small pieces.

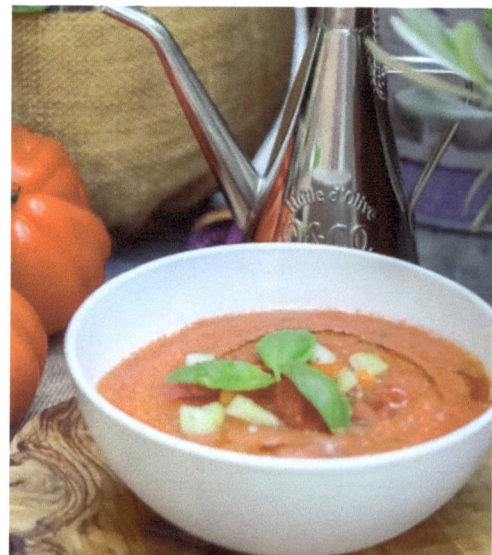

NUTRITIONAL VALUE | 1 serving (8oz.)
61 Calories; 3.4g Fat; 0 Cholesterol; 209.3mg Sodium; 7.1g Carbs - 1.4g Fiber, 5.9g Sugar; 1.5g Protein.

Sauces & Dippers

- Traditional Mexican Guacamole
- Pico de Gallo/Salsa
- Easy Hummus

POWER OF 5
Test Kitchen

Traditional Mexican Guacamole

We love avocados. Guacamole is a favorite to whip up at any time. Delicious on toast with cheesy veggie quesadillas or just plan with baked chips. Guacamole is easy to make and can be served at any meal!

PREP TIME 10 minutes

COOK TIME 0 minutes

PASSIVE TIME 0 minutes

SERVES 4

INGREDIENTS
- 2 avocados, peeled and pitted
- 1 cup chopped tomatoes
- Minced garlic
- 1/4 cup chopped onion
- 1/4 cup chopped cilantro
- 2 Tbsp lemon juice
- 1 jalapeño pepper, seeded and minced (optional)
- Salt and ground black pepper to taste

INSTRUCTIONS
1. Peel avocado, place in a bowl and mash until creamy.
2. Mix tomatoes, onion, cilantro, lemon juice, and jalapeño pepper into mashed avocado until well combined; season with salt and black pepper.

MELISSA'S MODIFICATIONS
If you want a purer avocado guacamole, omit the tomatoes chopped onions. Ingredients will include avocados, garlic, lemon juice, cayenne red pepper, salt and pepper, and cilantro if desired. Still very delicious.

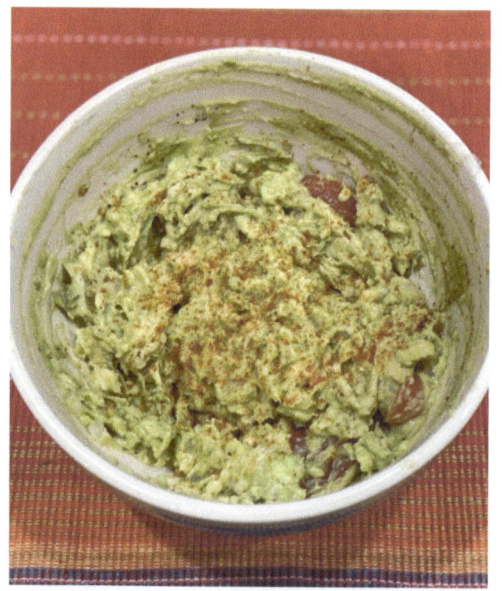

NUTRITIONAL VALUE | 1 serving
177 calories; protein 2.7g; carbohydrates 12.2g; fat 14.9g; sodium 49.9mg.

Pico de Gallo/Salsa

Pico de gallo or salsa is a delicious mix of Roma tomatoes, onions, lime juice, seasoning adding the heat of jalapeño peppers topped with cilantro. Served with chips—great for a starter or snack.

PREP TIME 20 minutes
COOK TIME 0 minutes
PASSIVE TIME 0 minutes
SERVES 12

INGREDIENTS
- 6 Roma (plum) tomatoes, diced
- 1/2 red onion, minced
- 3 Tbsp chopped fresh cilantro
- 1/2 jalapeño pepper, seeded and minced (optional)
- 1/2 lime, juiced
- 1 clove garlic, minced
- 1 pinch garlic powder
- 1 pinch ground cumin, or to taste
- Salt and ground black pepper to taste

INSTRUCTIONS
1. Chop the diced tomatoes and onions
2. Stir the tomatoes, onion, cilantro, jalapeño pepper, lime juice, garlic, garlic powder, cumin, salt, and pepper together in a bowl.
3. Refrigerate at least 3 hours before serving.

MELISSA'S MODIFICATIONS
Salsa is easy to make and can be used for an abundance of recipes. This is similar to the tomato mixture in bruschetta. I often use them interchangeably. The pico de gallo paired with chips and jalapeño vs. the bruschetta paired with olive oil and crusty bread—both use the same Roma tomatoes and seasonings!

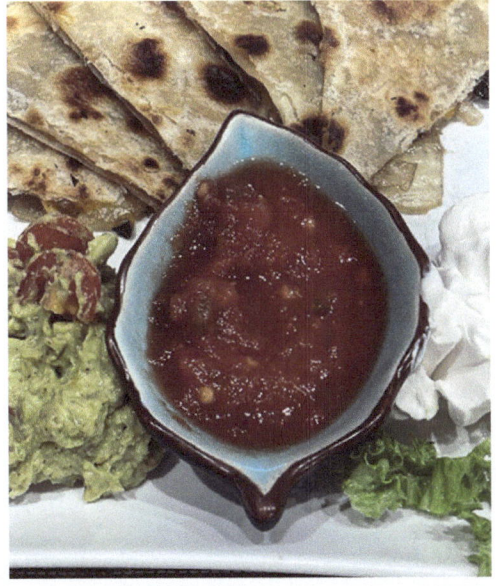

NUTRITIONAL VALUE | 1 serving
10 calories; protein 0.4g; carbohydrates 2.2g; fat 0.1g; sodium 15.2mg.

Easy Hummus

We love hummus! It is a delicious dip or spread made from chickpeas, tahini (sesame butter), lemon and spices. It is a Mediterranean and Middle Eastern favorite and is readily available in U.S. grocery stores. We prefer to make it at home as it is so easy to prepare!

PREP TIME	COOK TIME	PASSIVE TIME	SERVES
15 minutes	0 minutes	0 minutes	8

INGREDIENTS
- 1 15 oz can chickpeas
- 2 cloves garlic, peeled and minced
- 1 Tbsp tahini
- 1/4 cup lemon juice, freshly squeezed
- 1/4 tsp cumin
- 2 Tbsp extra-virgin olive oil
- Salt
- 2–3 Tbsp water, as needed for consistency
- Dash of paprika for serving

INSTRUCTIONS
1. Drain chickpeas, rinse well with cold water, set aside.
2. In the bowl of the food processor (or high-powered blender) – add the tahini and lemon juice, blend for 1 minute.
3. Scrape sides and bottom, then process for another 30 seconds.
4. Add olive oil, minced garlic, cumin and 1/2 tsp of salt to the tahini and lemon juice, continue to blend until creamy consistency.
5. Add half the drained chickpeas on low speed, blend well, then add the rest of the chickpeas. Add water, little at a time as needed to reach a smooth creamy consistency.
6. Add salt to taste.
7. Serve with drizzle of olive oil and a dash of paprika.

MELISSA'S MODIFICATIONS
If you are feeling ambitious and have the time, chickpeas can be homemade instead of from a can. If you have a pressure cooker or Instant Pot it is really quite simple. Soaked chickpeas usually take 12-14 minutes with natural release. Un-soaked chickpeas at high pressure with natural release takes 30-40 minutes. If you do not have a pressure cooker, you can soak the chickpeas overnight for beans to release. Delicious with pita chips, or any finger veggies such as carrots, celery, cauliflower or broccoli.

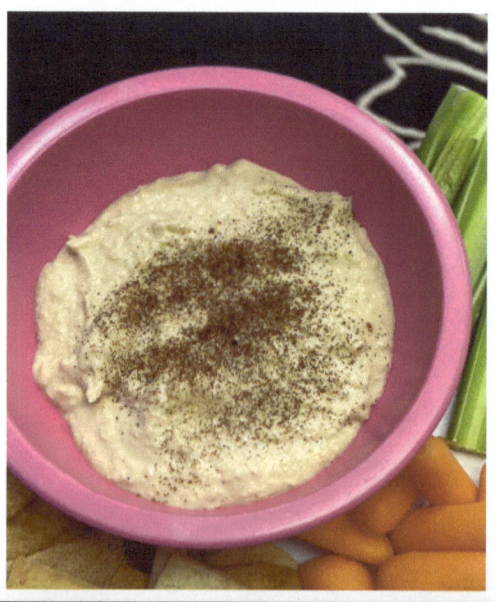

NUTRITIONAL VALUE | 1/4 cup serving, hummus only
190 Calories; 11g Fat; 18g Carbs - 5g Fibers, 3 g Sugars; 0 Cholesterol; 6g Protein

Main Dishes That Can Be Sides

- Cheese and Vegetable Quesadillas
- Stir Fry Veggies with Grilled Tofu
- Light Eggplant Parmesan
- Sheet Pan Fajitas
- BBQ Grilled Kebabs

POWER OF 5
Test Kitchen

Cheese and Vegetable Quesadillas

Quesadillas are a traditional Mexican dish with many variations based on cheese, vegetables, chicken, and/or combinations of all of these ingredients (see Melissa's Modifications below). Very easy to make in a stove top pan or in the oven. Great as a starter, lunch or dinner!

PREP TIME COOK TIME PASSIVE TIME SERVES

INGREDIENTS
- 2 tsp vegetable oil or vegan butter, divided
- 4 large flour tortillas (9- to 10-inch)
- 1–2 cups shredded cheese, such as cheddar, Monterey Jack, or any favorite melting cheese, low fat or vegan shredded cheese

FAVORITE FILLING COMBINATIONS
- Diced onion, mushrooms, diced red peppers, black beans, corn and cheddar
- Sautéed sliced mushrooms, shredded chicken breast, wilted spinach and Fontina
- Pulled pork, caramelized onions and Monterey Jack cheese
- Sautéed shrimp, red onion, avocado and queso fresco

INSTRUCTIONS
1. Melt 1/2 teaspoon butter or oil in the skillet. Ironically, the key to a crispy quesadilla is less fat in the pan, not more. Too much fat will make your quesadilla soggy instead of crispy. Use just enough to coat the bottom of your skillet — about 1/2 teaspoon of butter or oil. Warm it in the skillet over medium to medium-high heat.
2. Add the tortilla and top with cheese. Place 1 tortilla in the skillet and sprinkle all over with 1/2 cup of cheese.
3. Add the filling. Spread about 1/2 cup of filling in a single layer over just half the tortilla. Don't use too much or the filling will fall out as you try to eat it. Spreading the filling over half makes the quesadilla easier to fold, and adding it as the cheese melts gives the filling time to warm if it has cooled.
4. Watch for the cheese to melt. Once the cheese starts to melt, begin lifting a corner of the tortilla and checking the underside. When the cheese has completely melted and you see golden-brown spots on the underside of the tortilla, the quesadilla is ready.
5. Place another tortilla on the one cooking, wait a few minutes for the tortilla to stick, then with a large spatula, plate and cut in 4-6 pieces with a pizza cutter Or fold the quesadilla in half with a spatula.

Cheese and Vegetable Quesadillas

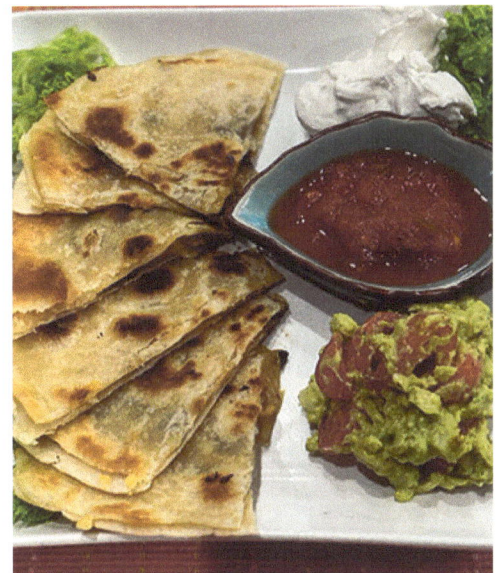

6. Transfer to a cutting board and cut into wedges. Slide the quesadilla onto a cutting board. If serving immediately, let cool for a minute or 2 for the cheese to set, then cut into wedges. If preparing several quesadillas for a crowd, slide the un-cut quesadillas onto a baking sheet and keep warm in a 200°F oven, then slice into wedges just before serving.
7. Wipe the pan clean if needed. Melt another dab of butter and continue cooking quesadillas as described above.

MELISSA'S MODIFICATIONS
Filling: leftover cooked vegetables, cooked meat, crumbled tofu, cooked beans, fresh or frozen corn, cooked rice or grains, or any other leftovers. Prepare the filling. Pick a few of the suggested filling ingredients above, enough to make 2 to 3 cups of total filling. If combining leftovers, warm them briefly in the microwave or in a skillet over medium heat. If using raw ingredients, cook before making quesadillas. Transfer the filling to a bowl and cover to keep warm.

Storage: Leftovers can be refrigerated in an airtight container for up to 5 days.

NUTRITIONAL VALUE | 1 serving (two stuffed tortillas)
280 Calories; 0mg Cholesterol; 690mg Sodium; 40g Carbs; 14g Fiber; 8g Protein

Stir Fry Veggies with Grilled Tofu

Stir fry is easy to prepare on the stove top or in a wok if you have one. It is very versatile as you can add vegetables, proteins, or even sauces of your choice. I like to keep it fresh and simple, with added grilled tofu as my protein. If desired, serve your stir fry over white or brown rice, ramen noodles, lo mein noodles, zoodles, or kale or spinach (my favorite for a base).

PREP TIME	COOK TIME	PASSIVE TIME	SERVES
20 minutes	30 minutes	0 minutes	6

INGREDIENTS

- 1 block of extra firm tofu, pressed and sliced
- 1 Tbsp olive oil
- 1 red bell pepper
- 1 yellow bell pepper
- 1 cup sugar snap peas
- 1 cup carrots, shredded
- 1 cup mushrooms, sliced
- 2 cups broccoli
- 2 cups of low-sodium soy sauce or Bragg Liquid Aminos for tofu bake and vegetables sauce
- 3 garlic cloves, minced
- 3 Tbsp brown sugar
- 1 tsp sesame oil
- 1/2 cup Better Than Bouillon vegetable broth (you can use chicken flavoring if you prefer)
- 1 Tbsp cornstarch
- 2 green onions, chopped for garnish (optional)
- Sprinkle of sesame seeds, for garnish (optional)

INSTRUCTIONS

1. Prepare tofu (or other protein of your choice).
2. Wrap block of tofu in a clean kitchen towel or paper towels to press out excess water.
3. Preheat oven to 400° F. Cover a sheet pan with parchment paper.
4. Slice pressed tofu in 1" slices and place on the sheet pan and brush with liquid aminos.
5. Bake for 10 minutes and then flip over for another 10 minutes.
6. Once tofu is slightly brown and done (careful not to overcook), pull out of oven and let cool for a few minutes.
7. Cut each slice into 3 or 4 slices. Put aside while you stir fry the vegetables.

Vegetable Stir Fry:

1. In a large skillet or a Wok, add 1 Tbsp olive oil over medium high heat.
2. Add vegetables of your choice: bell peppers, carrots, mushrooms, snap peas and broccoli. Sauté 3-5 minutes until veggies are almost tender.
3. In a small bowl, whisk together soy sauce or liquid aminos, garlic, brown sugar, sesame oil, broth, and cornstarch.
4. Pour over veggies and cook until the sauce has thickened.
5. Add in the cut tofu, and gently blend together.
6. Add chopped green onions and sesame seeds if desired.

Stir Fry Veggies with Grilled Tofu

MELISSA'S MODIFICATIONS

Stir fry is one of those dishes that is so versatile you can lend your creative juices. Optional vegetables can include asparagus, bean sprouts, celery, zucchini, cauliflower, onions, baby corn, water chestnuts, or other varieties of vegetables that you may desire. Almonds and cashews are great to stir in as well.

Add some heat by adding red chili sriracha sauce or crushed red pepper flakes.

You may replace the tofu with chicken or shrimp. If you do not add a protein, this will reduce the preparation time of the stir fry to 15 minutes!

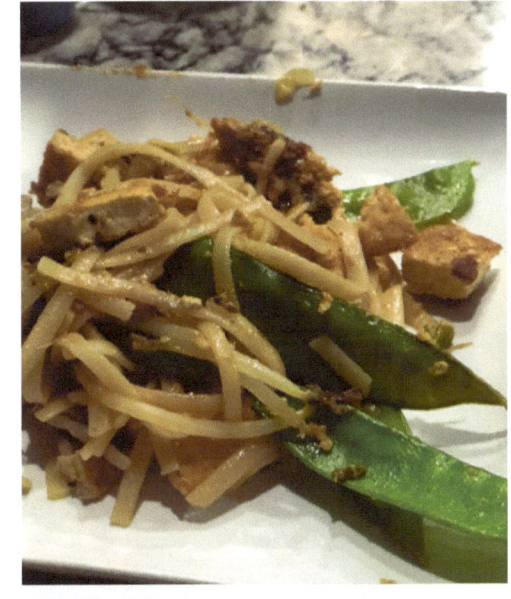

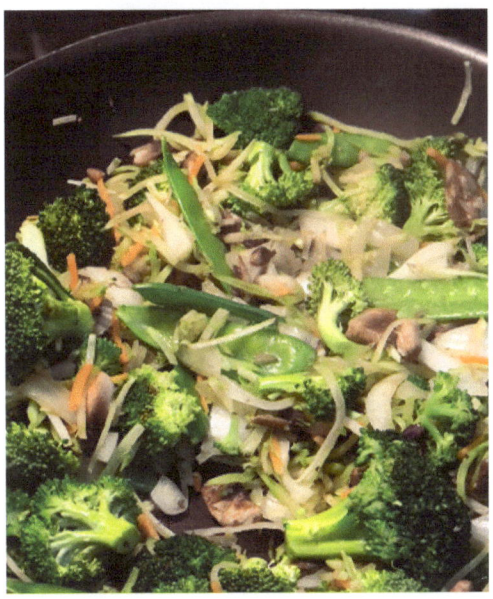

NUTRITIONAL VALUE | 1 serving with Tofu
274 Calories; 0mg Cholesterol; 6,541mg Sodium; 37.5 Carbs; 8.4g Fiber; 18g Protein

Light Eggplant Parmesan

Here is a lighter (and vegan) version of Melissa's Famous Eggplant Parmesan!
Still delicious, but lighter, fresh-tasting and even healthier.

PREP TIME	COOK TIME	PASSIVE TIME	SERVES
15 minutes	60 minutes	20 minutes	6

INGREDIENTS

- 2 medium eggplants, firm, good color, no bruise spots, sliced into 1/2"-1" pieces, leaving skin on as it helps keep shape and offers additional nutrition
- 1–2 Tbsp olive oil
- 1 8–10 oz jar organic tomato sauce
- Chopped garlic
- Part-skim mozzarella cheese (optional, substitute non-dairy cheese or do not use at all)
- Dried and crushed oregano
- Dried and chopped basil

Mushroom and Onion Sauté

- 1 medium to large sweet organic onion, peeled and chopped
- 8 oz mushrooms, cleaned and sliced
- 6 small organic Yukon Gold potatoes partially baked, then sliced
- 1–2 Tbsp Bragg Liquid Aminos for sauté and flavor
- Chopped garlic

INSTRUCTIONS

1. Slice eggplants to about 1/2" to 1" in thickness, leaving skin on. Salt the eggplants to remove any bitterness; rinse and dry over paper towels.
2. Preheat oven to 425° F. Prepare baking pans with parchment paper, coat by spraying with olive oil.
3. Since we are omitting the process of dipping in eggs and breadcrumbs, whisk the olive oil garlic and seasonings then cover the front and back of eggplant before baking. This will make a nice, crispy-on-the-outside, soft-on-the-inside eggplant.
4. Bake in the oven for 20 minutes in preheated oven. Flip over and bake another 20 minutes until both sides are nicely browned and a bit crispy.

Sauté Mushrooms, Onion and Potatoes:

1. In a medium sauce pan, sauté onions with the Braggs Liquid Aminos until the onions are almost lucid in color.
2. Add par-cooked potatoes to the onions and continue to sauté until all are nicely browned and cooked.
3. Add sliced mushrooms to the mix with pepper and other spices as desired until cooked.
4. Layer the cooked eggplant, tomato sauce, sautéed vegetables and cheese of your choice in a casserole and bake for 20 minutes until hot in 350° F oven.

Light Eggplant Parmesan

5. Alternatively, since all items are hot, you can skip the layering in a casserole step and plate layers directly for your guests. Sprinkle with Parmesan cheese (dairy or non-dairy) and serve right at the table.
6. Add salad and whole-grain breadsticks. Pair with a glass of red wine, and you're all set!

MELISSA'S MODIFICATIONS

I know this is different take on eggplant Parmesan, but if you wish to get closer to my original recipe, dip the eggplant into egg and breadcrumbs, if diet permits.

If you are following a vegetarian diet and eat dairy, you may dip the eggplant into egg whites before baking.

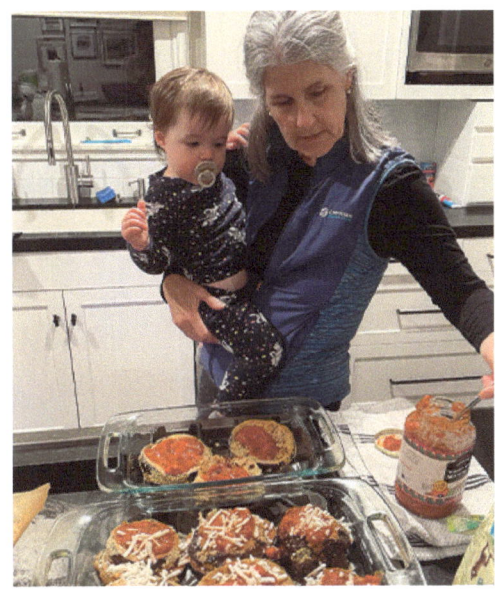

If you follow a plant-based vegan diet and want to bread the eggplants, I have used aquafaba (the liquid in canned chickpeas) or Just Eggs as the liquid in which to dip the eggplants. *A caution regarding breadcrumbs* ... read the labels as many have cheese in them. Be sure to get clean breadcrumbs with no dairy, especially if you are vegan.

Cook time – 40 minutes to bake the eggplant; 20 minutes on each side. If you bake the layered dish in the oven add another 20-25 minutes at 350° F.

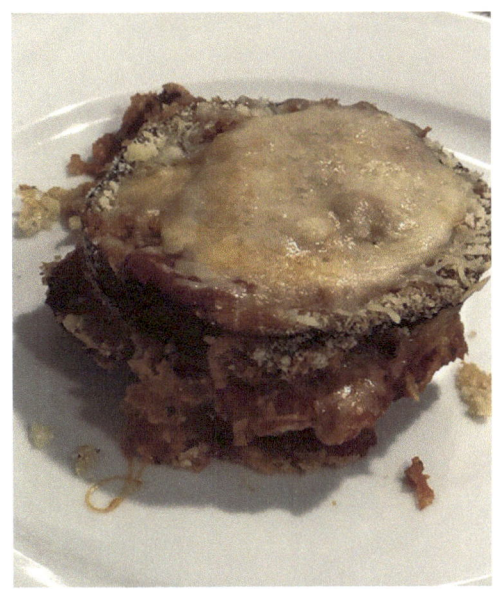

NUTRITIONAL VALUE | 1 serving
Calories 232, Carbs 22g(Fiber 8.4g), Protein 6g

Sheet Pan Fajitas

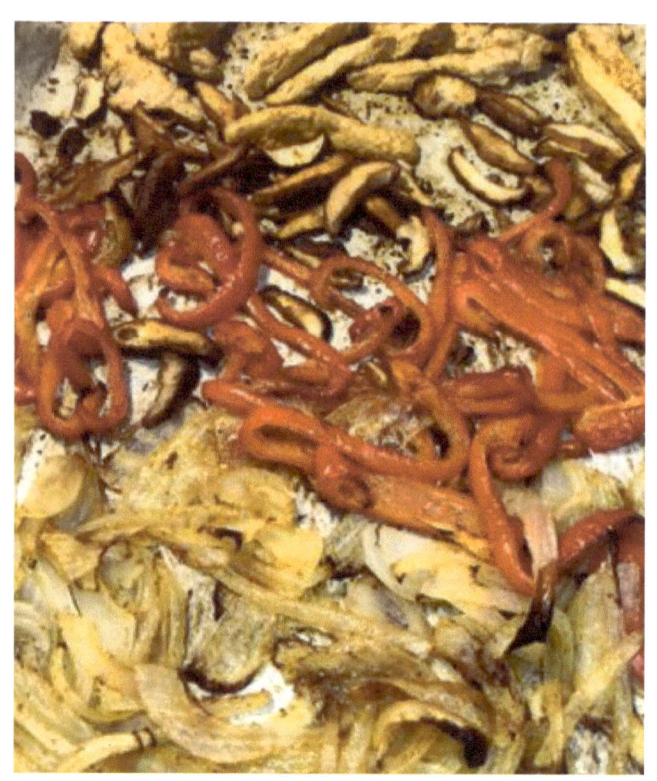
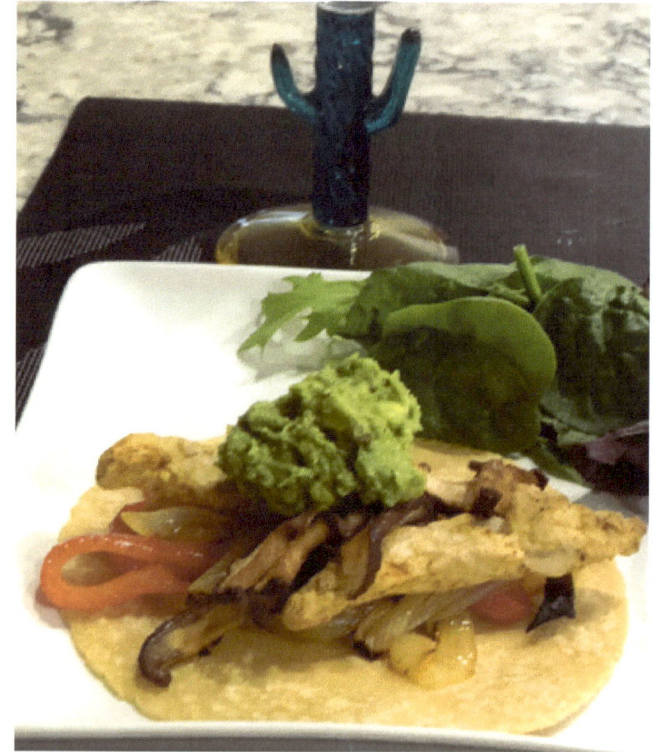

Sheet Pan Fajitas

An easy way to prepare all ingredients using only one pan!

PREP TIME
15 minutes

COOK TIME
20 minutes

PASSIVE TIME
0 minutes

SERVES
4

INGREDIENTS
- 1 package Gardein Chick'n Strips or 1.5 lbs of boneless, skinless chicken breasts sliced into 1/2-inch strips
- 1 green bell or red pepper sliced lengthwise
- 1 medium sweet onion, sliced
- 1/2 lb mushrooms, sliced (optional)
- 2 cloves garlic, minced
- 3 Tbsp olive oil
- 2 Tbsp lemon or lime juice
- 3 Tbsp chopped cilantro or parsley
- 8 taco sized tortillas flour or corn
- 1 cup sour cream, vegan or regular
- 1 cup guacamole, homemade or freshly-prepared store-bought
- 2 whole tomatoes, diced
- 2 tsp chili powder
- 1.5 tsp ground cumin
- 1 tsp paprika
- Salt and ground pepper to taste
- 1/2 tsp coriander
- Everything But The Bagel Seasoning to taste
- Sauté with water or Bragg Liquid Aminos (optional)

INSTRUCTIONS
1. Prep a 17"x12" sheet pan with parchment paper (my favorite), aluminum foil or just regular spray oil.
2. Preheat oven to 400° F.
3. For the seasoning: in a small bowl, whisk together chili powder, cumin, paprika, salt, and pepper. Set aside.
4. Slice peppers, onions and mushrooms. Place on the sheet pan.
5. If you are using fresh chicken (or if you are using plant-based Chik'n), place in a bowl. Add garlic, half of your oil, and half of the seasoning mixture, then stir together to coat the chicken.
6. Layer the seasoned and coated chicken on top of the vegetables in a single layer. If you are using pre-cooked Chick'n strips or plant-based coated chicken, wait to add to the sheet pan until the last fifteen minutes of baking as it is precooked.
7. After oven has preheated, roast the veggies and chicken, tossing halfway through. Bake until vegetables are fully cooked, about 20-25 minutes. If you used raw chicken, be sure it reaches 165° F in the center.
8. Warm tortillas by wrapping them tightly in aluminum foil and placing them in the warm oven for a few minutes.

MELISSA'S MODIFICATIONS
A fun and easy way to prepare dinner! Once done, you can even serve right from the pan. Other proteins can be used in place of plant-based options, such as shrimp or beef. Just be sure you gauge the cooking instructions based on the protein you choose to be sure the veggies and meats are fully cooked and the dish is ready to serve.

NUTRITIONAL VALUE | 1 serving
Calories 232, Carbs 22g(Fiber 8.4g), Protein 6g

BBQ Grilled Kebabs

Kebabs can be made with all kinds of meats, poultry and fish as well as all kinds of veggies, then grilled with a variety of sauces. Plan your kebab menu based on what you like. Kebabs can be one type of meat (of any type) or you can mix up kebabs with meats, veggies and fruit. There are no limits to what you can create. Sauces can vary depending upon the menu choice. I have chosen to grill using a homemade BBQ sauce that I use as a marinade prior to grilling.

PREP TIME	COOK TIME	PASSIVE TIME	SERVES
25 minutes	10 minutes	30 marinating time	8

INGREDIENTS

Main Ingredients

- 1 lb boneless chicken breasts, large shrimp, or beef tenderloin cut into to bite-sized pieces; if using shrimp, peel and devein, tails on or off
- 2 medium yellow and/or green zucchini cut into bite-sized pieces
- 1 large red onion, sliced and then cut into bite size pieces
- 2 large tomatoes, sliced into quarters so they are bite-sized, remove seeds

Homemade BBQ Sauce/Marinade

- 1 5.5 oz tomato paste (I use organic, but your choice)
- 2/3 cup apple cider vinegar
- 1 Tbsp white vinegar or lemon juice
- 2 Tbsp brown sugar or molasses
- 2 Tbsp mustard powder
- 1/4 cup maple syrup
- 2 Tbsp garlic powder
- 2 Tbsp smoked paprika
- 2 Tbsp sea salt
- 2 Tbsp fresh ground pepper
- 2 tsp natural raw sugar

INSTRUCTIONS

1. Sauce/marinade prepared first! Blend tomato paste, apple cider vinegar, maple syrup, molasses, mustard powder, garlic powder, smoked paprika, sea salt, ground black pepper, and sugar together in a blender.
2. Pour blended mixture into a saucepan and cook over medium heat, stirring constantly, until just heated through (about 5 minutes). Let cool for 10 minutes.
3. Combine the chicken or meat/shrimp (or all three!) and veggies together, coat well with some of the BBQ marinade in a bowl for 30 minutes. Keep rest of sauce separate for topping when serving.
4. Once the meat/shrimp is well marinated, begin to thread it, the zucchini, onion, and tomatoes onto the skewers.
5. Grill for 4–5 min per side or in the oven until the meat/shrimp is cooked. Beef will take a bit longer to cook to medium; shrimp will take less time.
6. Serve immediately with additional BBQ sauce if desired!

BBQ Grilled Kebabs

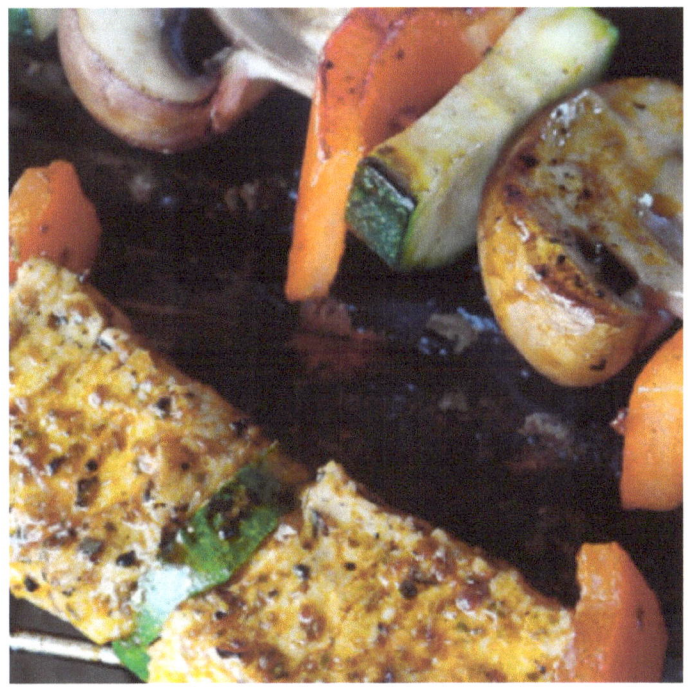

MELISSA'S MODIFICATIONS
If you are vegetarian or vegan, leave the meat out and add marinated tofu for protein, if desired.

Other options: the kebabs can be marinated veggies, or you can add fruit such as chunks of pineapple, peaches or watermelon ... delicious grilled! Add other veggies such as peppers, carrots, purple potatoes and corn ... be creative! Flavorings for marinating kebabs include seasonings and dipping sauces—endless! For sauces, think tahini, pesto, fruit glazes, teriyaki, Thai peanut, curry, or balsamic. Tossing skewer foods with olive oil and a seasoning such as za'tar, garlic, Italian spices, or Indian spices will add tons of flavors. Kebabs can be for dessert as well. Make a colorful fruit kebab by dipping in chocolate or other sweet sauces.

Enjoy being creative with kebab grilling! Use some of my suggestions or make up your own.

NUTRITIONAL VALUE | 1 serving Vegetable Kebabs - 84 Calories; 8.4g Carbs; 2.3g Fiber; 6.1g Sodium; 2.5g Protein. **Chicken Kebabs -** 200 Calories; 10.2g Fat; 26g Carbs; 4g Fiber; 31g Protein **Shrimp & Scallops -** 225 Calories; 15g Fat; 7g Carbs; 2g Fiber; 50mg Cholesterol; 14g Protein

Sides That Can Be Main Dishes

- Sheet Pan Roasted Green Beans and Baby Potatoes
- Elote – A Mexican Street Corn Dish
- Quinoa with Roasted Vegetables
- Roasted Italian Zucchini

POWER OF 5
Test Kitchen

Sheet Pan Roasted Green Beans and Baby Potatoes

Nothing brings out the flavor of vegetables like roasting them in the oven on a sheet pan!

PREP TIME
15 minutes

COOK TIME
20-30 minutes

PASSIVE TIME
0 minutes

SERVES
4

INGREDIENTS
- 1 lb bag baby potatoes, baby Dutch, purple, mixed – your choice
- 1 lb bag green beans, trimmed
- 2 Tbsp olive oil or olive oil spray
- 4 servings protein of your choice: roasted tofu, grilled chicken, shrimp, salmon
- 1–2 Tbsp garlic to taste
- Everything But The Bagel Seasoning to taste
- 3 cups organic beets, quartered, raw or par-cooked
- 1 Tbsp coconut oil

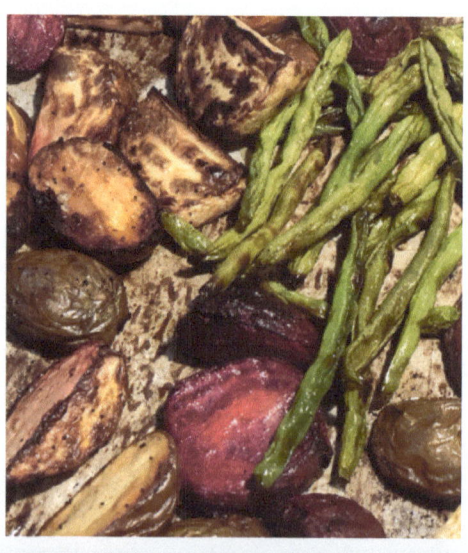

INSTRUCTIONS
1. Turn on the oven to the roast setting (if you have that setting) or pre-heat to 425° F.
2. Place parchment paper over your sheet pan (or you can use aluminum foil).
3. Cut potatoes in half and layer them on the pan. Spray with olive oil, then season with spices.
4. Since potatoes take a little longer than string beans to roast, give them a head start for about 8 minutes or so. If you add a dense vegetable, take this into account. For example, beets will take longer to cook if they are not parboiled.
5. Add the string beans after your more dense vegetables have baked. Roast until you have reached your preferred doneness. I like mine a bit on the crispier side.

Protein Choice Options
1. Season the protein of your choice. Depending on your choice, cooking times will vary. Add to the roasted vegetables.
2. Tofu: Roast based on firmness. I use firm and just roast on each side until nicely browned.
3. Chicken: Breasts can bake for 50–60 minutes, based on thickness.
4. Salmon: 6 – 8 minutes per side. Shrimp: 2–3 minutes per side.

MELISSA'S MODIFICATIONS
I have provided protein options within the recipe for your consideration. If you do not use oil, then you can coat the vegetables in your seasoning mixture after dipping them in vegetable broth. Just keep in mind different cooking times and temperatures to balance the sheet pan cook times.

NUTRITIONAL VALUE | 1 serving Vegetables (Baby Potatoes, Green Beans, Beets) only- 257 Calories; 7.4g Fat; 0 Cholesterol; 125.3mg Sodium; 33g Carbs; 11g Fiber; 6.6g Protein. **Added Protein - Tofu:** 173 Calories; 9g Fat;1g Carbs;8g Protein **Chicken Breast:** Without Skin - 119 Calories; 2.6g Fat; 61g Cholesterol; 53.6mg Sodium; 0g Carbs; 22.5g Protein **Salmon:** 4 oz. piece - 180 Calories;7g Fat; 57mg Cholesterol; 430mg Sodium; .1g Carbs; .5g Fiber; 22.1g Protein **Shrimp:** 9 pieces - 99 Calories; .3g Fat; 189mg Cholesterol; .2g Carbs; 24g Protein

Elote – A Mexican Street Corn Dish

This dish is nut, gluten, soy free. Very flavorful and makes a great side dish for summer cooking or grilling!

PREP TIME 20 minutes

COOK TIME 20 minutes

PASSIVE TIME 0 minutes

SERVES 6

INGREDIENTS

- 4 ears corn on the cob, can also use canned corn sautéed on the stove top until well-browned
- 2 Tbsp mayonnaise (If vegan, use Vegenaise or mayonnaise made with avocado oil.)
- 2 Tbsp sour cream (Non-dairy substitutes Tofutti®, Follow Your Heart, or Foragers® are all good.)
- 1 scallion, sliced
- 3/4 cups cotija cheese, crumbled (Feta cheese or Jack cheese can also be used. There are several vegan replacements. VioLife® is very close in taste. Vegan cheddar cheese works as well.)
- 1/4 tsp lime zest
- 1 Tbsp lime juice
- Pinch of chipotle chili powder
- 1/4 tsp sea salt

INSTRUCTIONS

1. Preheat your grill to medium-high.
2. Grill corn, turning occasionally, until highly charred and tender. About 8–12 min.
3. While the corn is grilling, in a medium bowl, whisk the mayo, sour cream, scallions, cheese, lime zest, lime juice and salt.
4. Once corn is grilled, let cool a bit before you cut the kernels off the cobs.
5. Add to the whisked mixture and toss to combined.

MELISSA'S MODIFICATIONS

This is a flavorful dish and is easy to prepare for those of you that do not eat dairy without loosing deliciousness. I have offered several replacement items to maintain the integrity of the dish.

Hope you try it ...
and love it like we do!

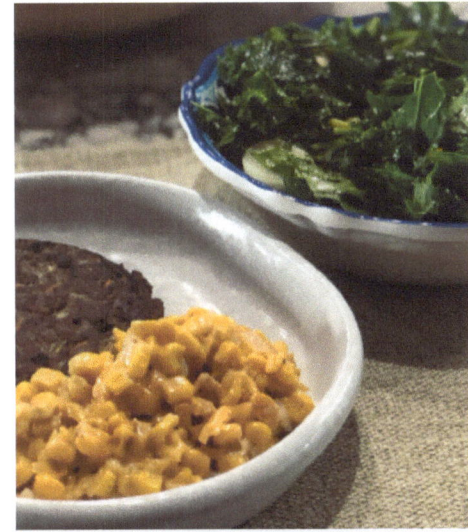

NUTRITIONAL VALUE | Per 1/2 serving 154 Calories; 13.9g Carbs; 9.6g Fat; 19mg Cholesterol; 348mg Sodium; 1.5g Fiber; 5g Sugar; 6g Protein. Additionally includes Vitamin C; Folic Acid; Calcium and Magnesium.

Quinoa with Roasted Vegetables

Easy and delicious recipe filled with protein, essential vitamins and amino acids.

PREP TIME	COOK TIME	PASSIVE TIME	SERVES
20 minutes	40 minutes	8 minutes	2

INGREDIENTS

Quinoa
- 1 cup quinoa, white, red, black or multi-mixed
- 1/2 tsp salt
- 3 cups water or 1 cup water plus 2 cups of vegetable broth
- 1/2 Tbsp olive oil, optional

Roasted Vegetables
- 1 4–6 oz package sweet peppers
- 1 medium onion, sliced
- 1 8 oz package mushrooms, sliced
- 2 Tbsp olive oil

INSTRUCTIONS

Quinoa
1. Rinse quinoa well
2. Put in a sauce pan with water/veggie broth and salt.
3. Bring to a boil then simmer for 15 minutes.
4. Quinoa will absorb the water/broth and change color to clear when it is done.

Roasted Vegetables
1. Turn oven temp for roasting to 425°F. Prepare roasting pan with parchment paper, add a thin layer of oil.
2. Prepare vegetables: wash, slice.
3. Spread veggies on roasting pan, sprinkle with salt and pepper and other seasonings you wish. I like to add garlic as well.
4. Sprinkle lightly with olive oil to coat veggies.
5. Roast for 25 minutes or so, turning several times during cooking time to get that beautiful roasted look on the sweet peppers and all vegetables are cooked.
6. Once vegetables are done, mix mushrooms and onions lightly into cooked quinoa. Place roated sweet peppers around quinoa in the serving platter.

MELISSA'S MODIFICATIONS
Feel free to use any vegetables or spices you wish when preparing this dish based on your likes.

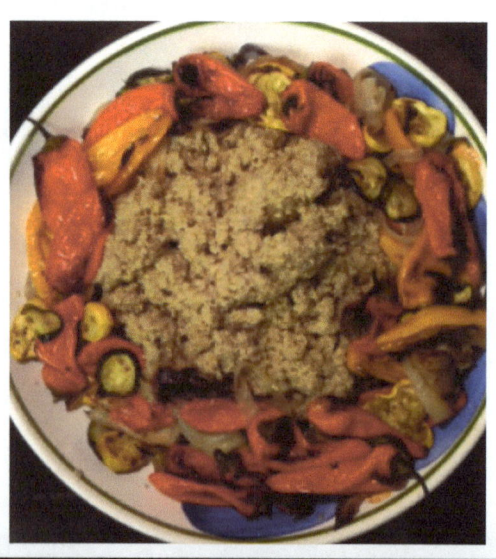

NUTRITIONAL VALUE | 1 serving
272 Calories; 8.9g Fat; 0g Cholesterol; 8.2mg Sodium; 21.8 Carbs - 3g Fiber; .7g Sugar; 5.2g Protein.

Roasted Italian Zucchini

Zucchinis are plentiful in the spring and through the summer. There are so many wonderful and tasty options—grilled, baked, sautéed or raw with a veggie dip!

PREP TIME
15 minutes

COOK TIME
30 minutes

PASSIVE TIME
5 minutes

SERVES
6

INGREDIENTS

- 4 nice-sized organic zucchini, washed, sliced lengthwise, about 3 slices per squash
- 1/2–3/4 cup mozzarella cheese, shredded (if you do not eat dairy, use an alternative such as Daiya® or Follow Your Healthy Heart®)
- 6 oz can organic tomato paste (alternatively, you can use tomato sauce)
- 5 – 6 pieces organic fire-roasted red peppers, sliced lengthwise (I buy Del-Destino brand of red peppers.)
- 2 cloves of fresh garlic, chopped
- 1 – 2 Tbsp basil, fresh or crushed
- 1 – 2 Tbsp oregano, crushed
- Himalayan pink salt to taste
- Pepper to taste
- Extra-virgin olive oil non-stick spray
- Everything But The Bagel Seasoning to taste (optional)

INSTRUCTIONS

1. Preheat oven to 375 °F. Prepare a lipped cooking pan with parchment paper. Spray with olive oil non-stick spray.
2. Clean zucchini and slice lengthwise. With a knife, lightly score width-wise across the zucchini, as this enhances cooking and helps toppings absorb! Layer on pan.
3. Spread tomato paste on the zucchini.
4. Layer red peppers on top of tomato paste, add basil, oregano, garlic and any other seasoning you may wish to add. I love Everything But the Bagel seasoning. It works great on these!
5. Sprinkle the mozzarella on top.
6. Cook on bake/roast setting on the middle rack of the oven for 20 minutes. Then move to the top rack on high broil for 5 minutes or so until the cheese is lightly browned. Watch carefully so they do not get too crispy!

MELISSA'S MODIFICATIONS

This is an easy and delicious recipe that can be used as a side dish, as I did with homemade spaghetti sauce and angel hair pasta. Add a piece of grilled fish or chicken along with a salad and you have a very healthy meal.

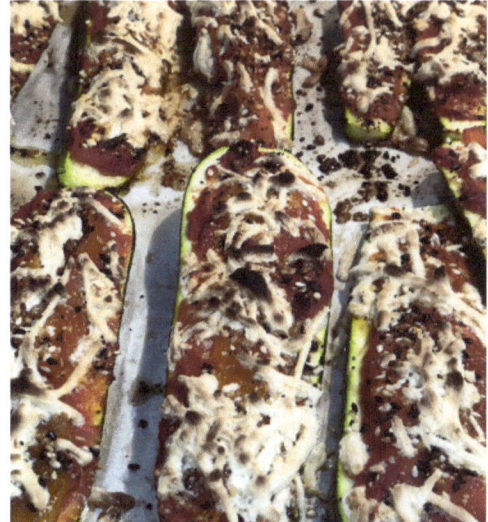

NUTRITIONAL VALUE | 1 serving
Calories 129, Protein 5.5g, Carbs 19g, Fiber 4.5g, Fat 3g.

Snacks Can Be Healthy

- Heart-Healthy Snacks
- Dr. B's Brain Health Trail Mix
- Grilled Fruit – Easy to Prepare and Delicious

POWER OF 5
Test Kitchen

Heart-Healthy Snacks

We are a snacking society! Staying away from the easy snacks like chips, candy and cookies is hard. They often give us momentary comfort. But comfort snack foods, which are often high in sugar, don't sustain our body's needs and do not feed a healthy heart. We can find satisfying heart-healthy snacks with careful consideration and some basic strategy. Kicking a sugar habit takes determination as sugar is an addiction substance. Removing sugar from your diet will allow you to taste the sweetness of fruits and vegetables like never before. Our go-to snacks include mixed berries, apples, celery with nut butter, or a hand full of raw, unsalted nuts. Reading labels is a must, and be cautious of portion size.

PREP TIME	COOK TIME	PASSIVE TIME	SERVES
15 minutes	10 minutes	0 minutes	1

GO-TO HEART HEALTHY SNACK SUGGESTIONS

- Carrots with hummus (See hummus recipe in Sauces & Dippers chapter)
- ¼ cup mixed unsalted and raw nuts or seeds
- NuttZo® 7 Nuts & Seeds Power Fuel Butter (If you have a peanut allergy, this nut and seed butter is for you as it does not contain peanuts! No added sugar, Paleo and vegan friendly.)
- Whole-grain rice cakes with nut butter and ½ banana
- Fresh sliced apples with nut butter
- Celery with a nut butter
- Whole-grain rice cakes with sliced avocados sprinkled with Everything But The Bagel seasoning
- Hearts of Palm, eat right out of the jar (SunPix brand from Costco)
- Orange and grapefruit slices
- Fresh berry fruit salad

MELISSA'S MODIFICATIONS

You cannot go wrong with any of these snacks as long as you maintain portion control.

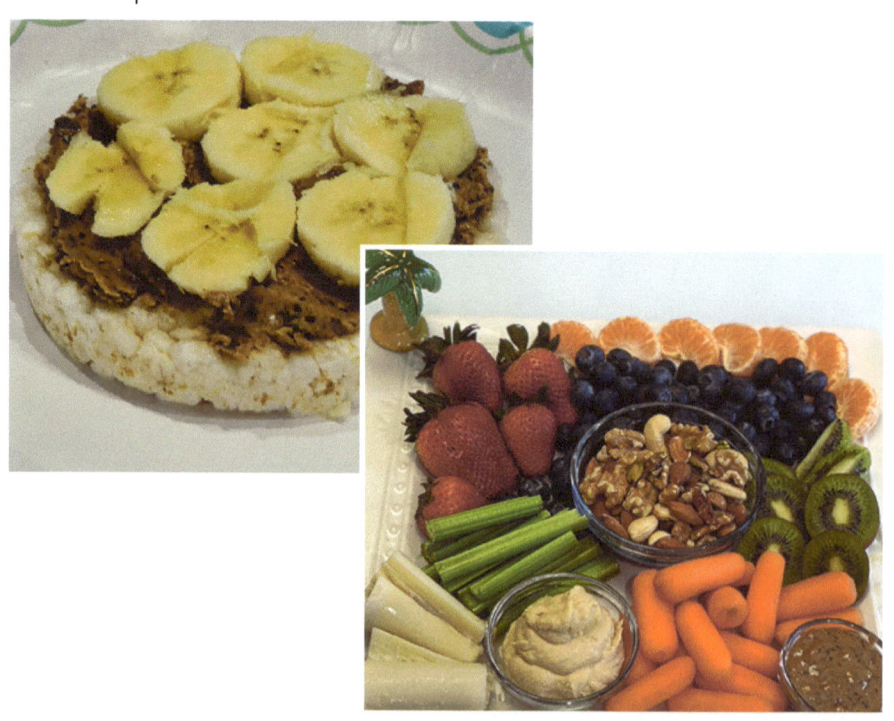

NUTRITIONAL VALUE | **Mixed unsalted Nuts:** 1/4 cup Serving: 170 Calories; 7g Carbs; 2g Fiber; 15g Fat; 0 Cholesterol; 5g Protein. **Homemade Hummus:** 1/4 cup Serving - 190 Calories; 18g Carbs; 5g Fibers; 11g Fat; 0 Cholesterol; 6g Protein. **Carrots & Celery with Nut Butter:** Celery & Carrots Free Foods! The added Nut Butter is your added nutrition. 180 Calories; 8g Carbs; 3g Fiber; 15g Fat; 0 Cholesterol; 6g Protein. **Mix Berries Fruit Salad:** 2 cups - 160 calories; 40g Carbs -11g Fiber, 29g Natural Sugar; 3g Protein

Dr. B's Brain Health Trail Mix

A delicious and nutritious snack for your brain and heart with ingredients that are anti-inflammatory and are anti-inflammatory and contain probiotics. They provide a good base for a healthy pick-me-up energy snack.

PREP TIME	COOK TIME	PASSIVE TIME	SERVES
15 minutes	30 minutes	0 minutes	8-10

INGREDIENTS

- 1 cup cashews, raw and unsalted
- 1 cup almonds, raw and unsalted
- 1 cup walnuts, raw
- 1/2 cup pistachios, unsalted and shelled
- 1/2 cup pumpkin seeds, raw
- 1/2 cup sunflower seeds, raw
- 1/2 cup dried blueberries
- 1/2 cup raisins
- 1/2 cup dark chocolate, 70% or higher (Ghirardelli® 60% dark chocolate chips will do too.)
- 1 tsp turmeric
- 1/2 tsp kosher salt
- 2 tsp curry powder
- 1 – 2 Tbsp coconut oil
- 2 tsp maple syrup
- 1/2 tsp fresh ground pepper
- 1/4 tsp cayenne pepper

INSTRUCTIONS

1. Preheat oven to 350°F.
2. Line baking sheet with parchment paper.
3. Combine the cashews, almonds, walnuts, pistachios, pumpkin and sunflower seeds in a mixing bowl.
4. In a small bowl, combine the curry powder, turmeric, kosher salt and ground pepper.
5. Sprinkle over the nuts and toss to combine.
6. Drizzle the coconut oil and maple syrup over the nut mixture. Blend until the nuts are evenly coated.
7. Spread the mixture onto the prepared baking sheet.
8. Bake, stirring once, until nuts are golden brown, about 35–40 minutes.
9. Let cool on the baking sheet.
10. Once cooled, store in an airtight container.
11. If it lasts this long, it can last up to 3 days in room temperature. (Ours was gone in 2!)

MELISSA'S MODIFICATIONS

Dr. B. had fun making this trail mix and adding his own blend and touches. The nuts are flexible – if you are not fond of a nut, substitute for another one. Brazil nuts are another option to substitute. Same applies with the seeds. They are optional or switch them out.

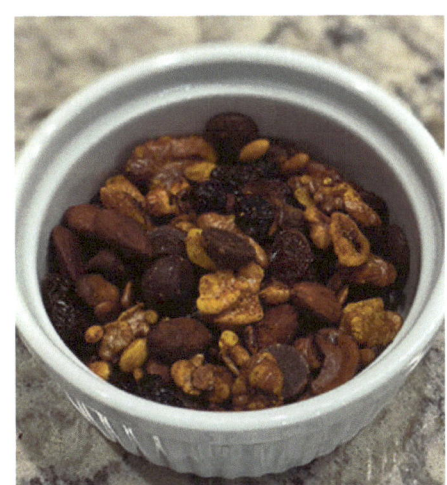

NUTRITIONAL VALUE | 1 serving (2oz)
486 Calories; 49.9 Fats(healthy); 0 Cholesterol; 9.2mg Sodium; 43.9 Carbs - 8.6g Fiber; 17.5 Sugars; 25g Protein

Grilled Fruit – Easy to Prepare and Delicious

Grilled fruit is a great appetizer, side dish or dessert. The amounts you grill will vary based on the number of people you are serving.

PREP TIME	COOK TIME	PASSIVE TIME	SERVES
30 minutes	15 minutes	0 minutes	4

INGREDIENTS
- 1 whole pineapple, cut off the top and heel then trim off the sides (leave the core in if you wish or remove it)
- 4 peaches, sliced in half and pitted
- 2 bananas, slice lengthwise and leave peel on while grilling (the more ripe the better!)
- Cinnamon and sugar

INSTRUCTIONS
1. Take any fruit you wish to grill and prepare for grilling. Clean, cut and pit.
2. If your grill has two heating stations, then start with grilling on the hot side so you get the nice grill look. As it cooks move to the lower heat section for thorough cooking.
3. Pineapple: Grill until it has nice grill marks and the surface is slightly caramelized. Flip and grill the other side, then move to the lower heat until they are slightly tender but not too soft.
4. Peaches: Place half of the peaches cut side down on the grill. Cook until they have good grill marks or are slightly caramelized. Move them to the lower heat side of the grill to finish up or until they become more tender, but not too soft. If using for dessert, sprinkle a little cinnamon sugar on the cut grilled side.
5. Bananas: Grill the bananas cut-side down, skin-side up. Once there is a slight grill mark, move carefully to the cooler grill side so they can heat through, not getting burnt or get too soft. Once tender, move from the grill and sprinkle with cinnamon sugar.

MELISSA'S MODIFICATIONS
Enjoy these easy-to-grill fruits of your choice, following the same simple grilling methods as stated above. This is a refreshing low-calorie alternative for appetizers, side dishes or desserts. If you don't grill, use the broil feature in your oven!

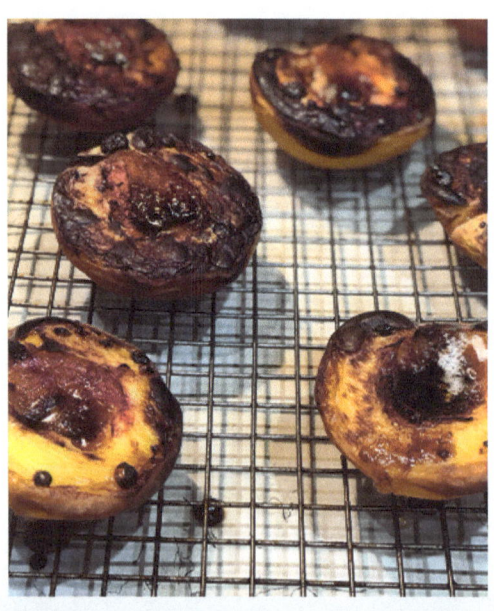

NUTRITIONAL VALUE |
Grilled Peaches- 2 halves = 95 Calories; Fat 1.5g; Carbs 16g (Fiber 2g ; Sugars 14g); Protein 5g

Yes ... Healthy Desserts Please!

- Non-Dairy Frozen Fruits Ice
- Oatmeal Fruit Bake
- Berries Yogurt Parfait with Dark Chocolate Drizzle
- Homemade Applesauce with Strawberries

POWER OF 5
Test Kitchen

Non-Dairy Frozen Fruits Ice

Delicious, refreshing alternative to a common dessert staple.

PREP TIME
10 minutes

COOK TIME
0 minutes

PASSIVE TIME
5 minutes

SERVES
4

INGREDIENTS
- 6 bananas, sliced and frozen for at least 1 day
- 1 Tbsp vanilla
- 1/2 cup soy or almond milk

INSTRUCTIONS
1. Purée the frozen bananas in a food processor or Magic Bullet.
2. Add vanilla and soy or almond milk and blend until smooth.
3. Pour into a large bowl and serve immediately.

MELISSA'S MODIFICATIONS
You can add strawberries to the bananas for additional flavor or make a strawberry and apple ice cream using vanilla and soy or almond milk. For additional sweetness, add a tsp of maple syrup. Add a Tbsp of vanilla protein powder for added thickness.

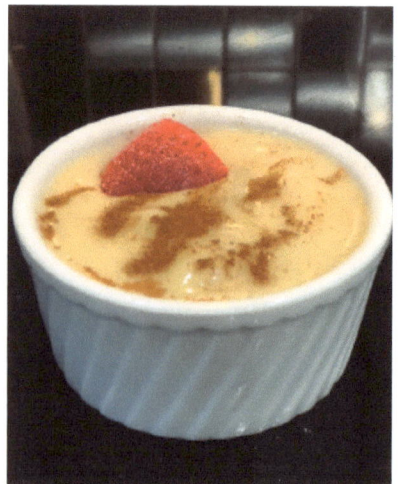
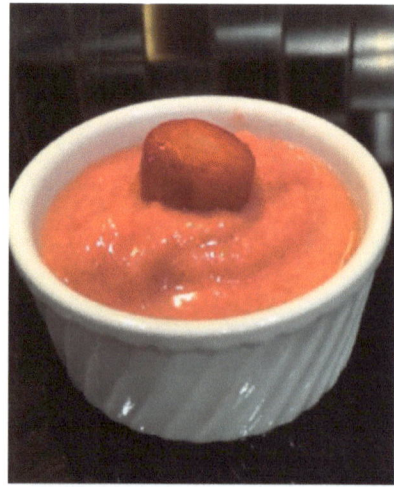

NUTRITIONAL VALUE | 1 serving (approx 1.5 cups) *Banana*: Calories 123 per serving; Protein 2.9g; Carbs 24.1g (3.6g Fiber, 12.4g Sugar)
Strawberry/Apple with protein powder: Calories 218 per serving;Protein 2.4g, Fat 2.2g ; total carbs 37.5g (7.5g Fiber, 26g sugar)

Oatmeal Fruit Bake

A moist and fruit-filled oatmeal bake. Make two batches and freeze one for the future!

PREP TIME
15 minutes

COOK TIME
60 minutes

PASSIVE TIME
5 minutes

SERVES
6

INGREDIENTS

- 2 cups old fashioned rolled oats
- 1/4 cup 100% maple syrup (alternative, use 6-8 drops of stevia extract)
- 1 tsp baking powder
- 1 tsp cinnamon
- 1/2 tsp sea salt
- 2 cups almond milk
- 1 large egg or 3 Tbsp of "Just Eggs" or 1 Tbsp ground flaxseed
- 2 Tbsp organic coconut oil (expelled, pressed and refined—there is no coconut taste)
- 2 tsp pure vanilla extract
- 2 ripe bananas, mash one banana to add to the oatmeal mixture and slice one for the top
- 1–2 cups fresh strawberries, sliced, save 1/4 cup for the top of the fruit bake
- 1/4 cup dark chocolate chips, add 1/2 into the mixture and sprinkle half on top (optional)
- 1 cup blueberries

INSTRUCTIONS

1. Preheat oven to 375°F.
2. Line square baking dish with parchment paper or spray glass baking dish with cooking spray.
3. In a large bowl, mix oats, baking powder, cinnamon, and salt.
4. Add in almond milk, maple syrup, egg (or egg substitute), coconut oil, vanilla, and mashed banana. Stir well to combine all the ingredients.
5. Gently fold in 1 cup of strawberries and blueberries as well as 1/2 of the bananas.
6. Bake in oven for about 55 minutes, until it bubbles and looks like the middle has set. Should be golden brown on the edges.
7. Remove from oven, and let it sit for a bit to cool down and set some more.

MELISSA'S MODIFICATIONS

This recipe offers so much variation! Use other fruits and berries—your choice. The dark chocolate chips are optional but add deliciousness, especially if you are enjoying as a dessert. To reduce the sugar and calories, use 6–8 drops of stevia extract (or similar sweetener*). You could even leave out the sweetener as the fruit may supply enough sugar for your taste.

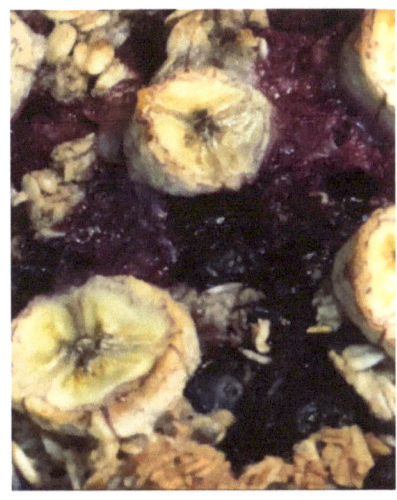

NUTRITIONAL VALUE | 1 serving 286 Calories (251 calories, if you use stevia or similar replacement); 8.5g Fat; 142g Sodium; 0 Cholesterol; 40g Carbs (*32.5g if using stevia extract); 6g Fiber; 17g Sugar (*9.7g if using stevia extract); 6g Protein. **If you add the dark chocolate chips:** 60% Ghirardelli Chocolate Chips: 20g (1/4c) = 302 calories (50c per servicing) 22.7g Fat; 26g Carbs; 3.8g Fiber; 22.7g Sugar; 3.8g Protein.

Berries Yogurt Parfait with Dark Chocolate Drizzle

An easy and delicious dessert that is light and a perfect end of any meal.
Best made in individual cup servings for presentation.

PREP TIME	COOK TIME	PASSIVE TIME	SERVES
15 minutes	0 minutes	0 minutes	4-6

INGREDIENTS

- 8–12 oz yogurt, plain, vanilla or non-dairy yogurt
- 2 cups mixed berries of your choice
- 1 tsp vanilla, if using plain yogurt
- Several drops Stevia Clear, if more sweetening is needed for plain yogurt
- 2 oz melted dark chocolate chips (I prefer Ghirardelli® Brand—60% Cacao)

INSTRUCTIONS

1. Wash and dry berries of your choice, hull and cut strawberries into pieces, keep a few fresh uncut strawberries for garnish.
2. If you are using plain yogurt, place it in a bowl and add pure vanilla and Stevia Clear to get the right flavor.
3. Use 8 oz parfait glass or plastic 8 oz wine glass to assemble the ingredients.
4. Spoon the yogurt mixture into the bottom of each of the parfait glasses, then add a layer of berries, then more yogurt, berries … repeat until you reach the top.
5. Slice the whole strawberry so you can hook onto the top of the glass for presentation.
6. Melt the dark chocolate in the microwave or in a double boiler.
7. Drizzle the dark chocolate over the top of the fruit & yogurt parfait and serve.

MELISSA'S MODIFICATIONS

This is an easy dessert and very fun to eat. If you make ahead of time, you can refrigerate until ready for dessert, then prepare the dark chocolate and drizzle while hot … very delicious.

Healthy granola that is lightly sweetened with honey can also be one of the layers in your parfait.

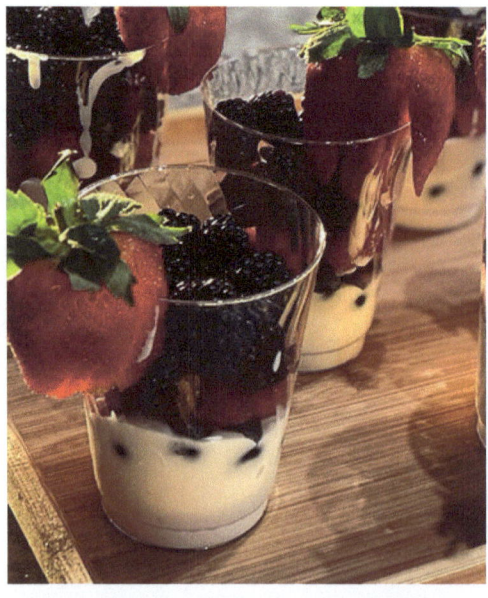

NUTRITIONAL VALUE | 1 serving
140 calories;8g Fat; 14.5g Carbs- 3g Fiber, 11.3g Sugar; 4g Protein.

Homemade Applesauce with Strawberries

After eating my homemade applesauce with strawberries, my husband raved it was "award-winning!" I'm not sure about that, but it was delicious! Try it and see what you think!

PREP TIME	COOK TIME	PASSIVE TIME	SERVES
15 minutes	10 minutes	0 minutes	4-6

INGREDIENTS

- 4 – 6 medium organic apples, cored and cut into chunks
- 8 – 10 oz package organic frozen whole strawberries
- 1/2 cup water
- 1-2 tsp light agave sweetener (or to taste)
- 2 tsp cinnamon (or to taste)
- Walnuts or almonds (optional)

INSTRUCTIONS

1. Wash, core and cut apples into chunks. I leave the skin on, you may remove when you are preparing the apples if you wish.
2. Pour the water in a medium pan and bring to a boil. Throw the apples in and when it begins to boil again, reduce the heat, cover and let cook. Check often and stir.
3. When apples are almost done, add strawberries and continue to cook covered for 6–8 minutes until all fruits are soft and well-blended.
4. Add agave (or your choice of sweetener), spices and stir well into applesauce.
5. Remove from heat and keep covered so the agave and cinnamon can absorbed and blend with the fruits.
6. Refrigerate once cooled. Enjoy!

MELISSA'S MODIFICATIONS

For this easy to make recipe, I used Braeburn apples. Honey Crisp apples are also good, sweet and delicious. You can use fresh strawberries or other berries as well to add flavor and variety. Add nuts on the top when servicing with a little extra cinnamon. To skin or not to skin? I always include the skin when I cook a recipe with apples because of the nutritional value. The skin is loaded with it! The skin of one apples contains 5 mg of fiber, 13 mg of calcium, 239 mg of potassium, and 10 mg of vitamin C. The skin is not to be missed with all that nutrition—that is why I only buy organic apples and strawberries (and all fruits and vegetables) so I worry less about harmful pesticide residue.

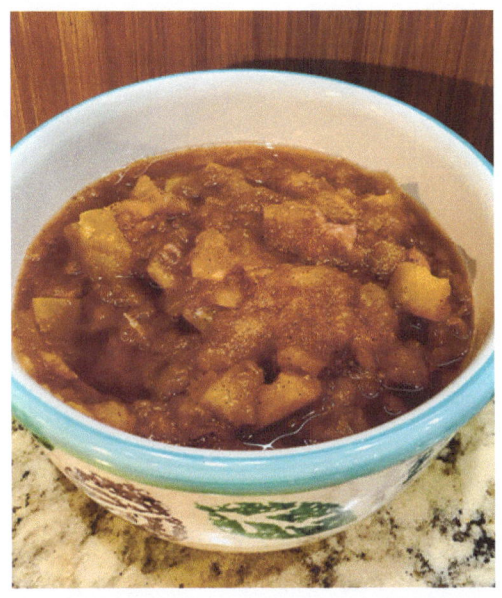

NUTRITIONAL VALUE | 1 serving
Calories 232, Carbs 22g(Fiber 8.4g), Protein 6g

Closing Tastes: Thoughts from Melissa

I hope you enjoy the recipes and suggestions provided in the Power of 5 Test Kitchen Cookbook—Caregiver Edition. Caregivers play such an essential role for those in their care. I applaud your strength and willingness to take on a difficult challenge.

Encouraging participation and engagement on a daily basis may be trying and exhausting. Taking small bite-sized steps, starting with a simple recipe when you begin cooking is the key to a safe and meaningful activity. I hope you both will be pleasantly surprised at how fulfilling a cooking activity can be, especially if you take it slow, step by step, and have fun in the process!

Resources

The following resources are a guide to promote a safe and meaningful experience in the kitchen, as well as providing healthy and nutritious meals to those who have a neurodegenerative disorder.

Healthy Eating on a Daily Basis

As I mentioned earlier, eating for your health is very important for everyone and especially for anyone fighting a disease and especially when cooking for individuals with neurodegenerative disease. **Research has shown that a diet high in protein, low in carbohydrates, and with little or no sugar** provides the most favorable outcomes.

The following table-setting diagrams in this section will provide some guidance and guidelines, along with two lists: unlimited vegetables and healthy carbohydrates. Also ... don't forget to drink plenty of water throughout the day! These eating guides are from Dr. Bernstein's book, *The Power of 5: The Ultimate Formula for Longevity & Remaining Youthful* on pages 177–181. They are gratefully included with permission.

Healthy Eating on a Daily Basis

BREAKFAST

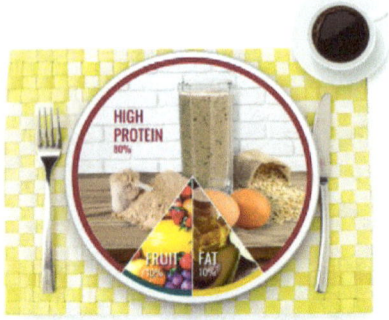

75 – 80% protein: egg recipe, shake or oatmeal with protein powder
10% fat: avocado, nuts
10 – 15% fruit
Non-caloric beverage: tea or coffee without sugar or artificial sweetener

LUNCH

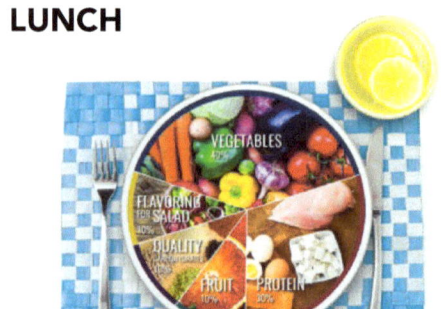

40% vegetables
30% protein
10% fruit
10% quality carbohydrates: grains, quinoa, beans or legumes
10% flavoring for salads or vegetables

DINNER

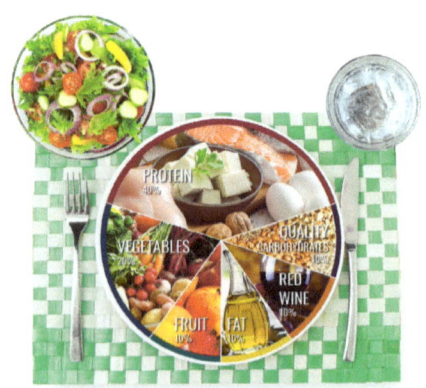

20% vegetables
40% protein
10% fruit
10% quality carbohydrates: grains, quinoa or legumes
10% fat: olive oil, avocado, etc.

Unlimited Vegetables — Enjoy up to 2 cups for lunch and dinner

- Artichokes
- Arugula
- Asparagus
- Beans, yellow or green
- Beets
- Bell Peppers
- Bok Choy
- Broccoli
- Brussels sprouts
- Cabbage
- Carrots
- Cauliflower
- Celery
- Chili peppers
- Collard greens
- Cucumbers
- Endive
- Eggplant
- Escarole
- Fennel
- Garlic
- Ginger
- Jicama
- Kale
- Leeks
- Lettuce
- Mushrooms
- Okra
- Onions
- Peas
- Peppers
- Radish
- Snow peas
- Spinach
- Sprouts
- Squash
- Tomato
- Turnips
- Watercress
- Zucchini

Healthy Carbohydrates — Portion size 1/4 cup per day is preferred

GRAINS
- Amaranth
- Buckwheat groats (kasha)
- Brown rice
- Millet
- Quinoa
- Teff (grain from Ethiopia)
- Wild rice

VEGETABLES
- Corn
- Squash-summer and winter varieties
- Sweet potatoes
- Water chestnuts

BEANS
- Black beans
- Chickpeas (garbanzo beans)
- Great northern beans
- Kidney beans
- Lentils
- Lima beans
- Navy beans
- Pinto beans
- Soy milk
- Soy yogurt
- Soybeans and edamame
- Split peas
- Tofu
- White beans (cannellini)

This **Abilities Inventory** will assist you in determining the level of abilities of the individual before a cooking activity and to explore likes/dislikes. It is a guide to keep cooking activities appropriate for the level of the individual.

Purposeful Engagement through Food & Meal Preparation (PEMP) for the Caregiver and Those in Their Care with Neurodegenerative Disorders

Abilities Inventory for Cooperative Cooking Activity

Melissa C. Bernstein, OT, FAOTA

Instructions: Complete this skills inventory with the individual prior to a cooking activity. *Mark in non-shaded areas.*

Name: _____

Functional Abilities	Yes/No	Good	Fair	Poor
Standing Balance				
Standing Tolerance				
Sitting Tolerance				
Attention span				
Vision				
Glasses				
Hearing				
Hearing Aids				
Hand Strength				
Hand Grasp				
Fine Motor Skills				
Upper Extremity Strength				
Using Hand/Arms Together				
Comments:				

ADLs, IADLs	No Assist Needed	Some Assist	Complete Assist	Not Applicable
Meal Preparation				
Meal Planning				
Cooking				
Clean-Up				
Storage of Food				
Ability to Safety Use Kitchen Equip & Utensils				

Cooking Skills Abilities	No Assist Needed	Some Assist	Complete Assist	Not Applicable
Washes Hands before meal prep				
Safety handles knives & other implements				
Can preheat the oven & use pot holders for safety				
Turns off stove after use				
Can follow a recipe				
Can prepare ingredients from a recipe				
Follows proper table manner				
Food preparation				
Thaws frozen food in time for meal prep				
Familiarity with safe handling practices & risk of cross contamination				
Washes fruits & veggies before cooking & eating				
Kitchen Cleanup				
Cleans prep dining area before/after eating				
Scrapes, rinses and places dirty dishes in diswasher after eating				
Loads dishwasher				
Store clean dishes in designated areas				
Store food in covered, sealed containers				

Foods Likes & Dislikes Inventory

Questions	Responses
What are your favorite foods?	
Do you have any food allergies?	
Fruits? What type?	
Vegetables What type?	
Bread? What type?	
Meats?	
Poultry?	
Fish?	
Desserts?	
What is your favorite meal? Why?	
Comments:	

Completed by: _____ Date: _____

Adaptive Kitchen Equipment

These include some basics that are available on Amazon or other (DME) durable medical equipment stores to provide resources that may be utilized to promote independence. For further guidance regarding the best adaptive pieces of equipment to use, contact an occupational therapist for assistance if needed.

NOTE: Information and photos used from Amazon site are for examples for purchase by the companies listed.

Adaptive Eating Utensils

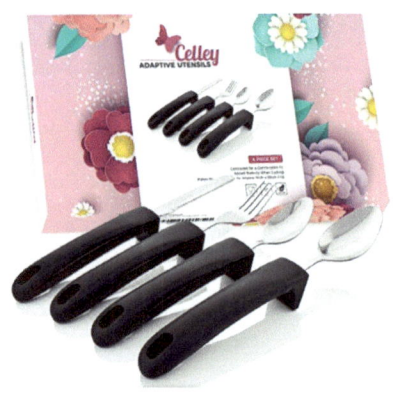

Adaptive Eating Utensils by Celley for Parkinson's, Arthritis, MS, Elderly, Hand Tremors, Handicapped 4pc Easy Grip Silverware Stainless Steel Knife, Fork, 2 Spoons – (Black)

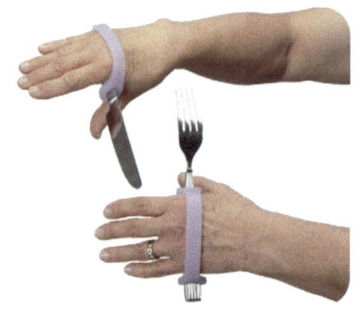

CrazyHold Silicone Adaptive Aid (12 Years to Adults) for individuals with Limited Hand Mobility, Cerebral Palsy, Stroke—Perfect for occupational therapy or physical therapy use (Lavender - 5 1/4")

Adaptive Kitchen Equipment

Adaptive Eating Utensils

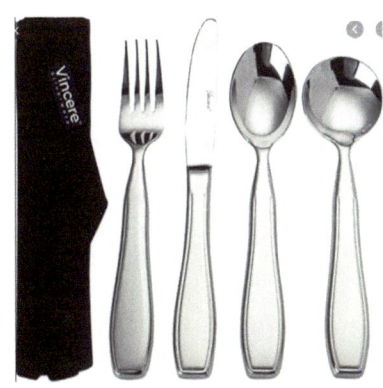

Weighted Utensils for Tremors and Parkinson's Aids Devices - Heavy Weight Stainless Steel Silverware Set, Adaptive Eating Flatware Helps Hand Tremors, Parkinson, Arthritis - Knife, Fork, 2 Spoons & Bag

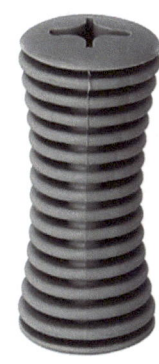

SP Ableware Universal Built-Up Handle (Pack of 4) (746300000)

Adaptive Kitchen Equipment

Adaptive Cutting Boards

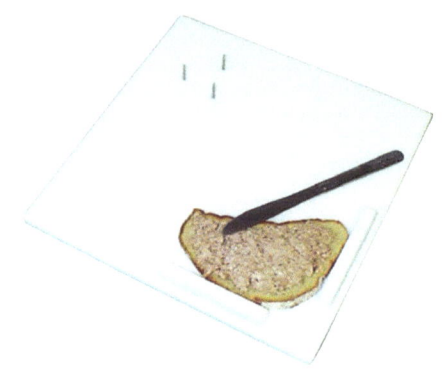

Parsons ADL 61-0200 Cutting Board, 12" x 12"

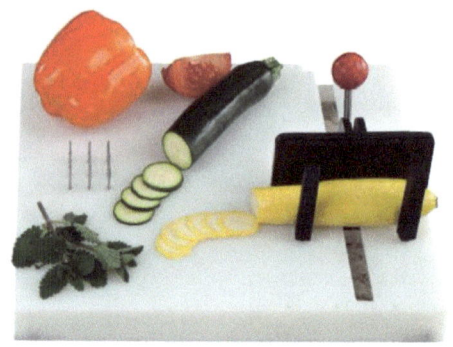

Etac Deluxe One-Handed Paring Board With Rocker Knife

Safety Knives

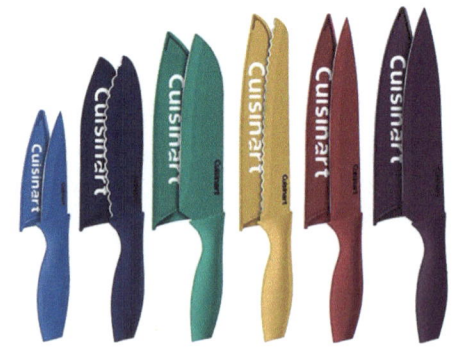

https://www.cuisinart.com/shopping/cutlery/advantage_sets/c55-01-12pcks/

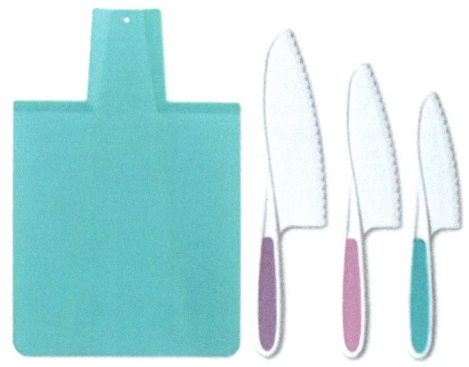

Tovla Jr Kids Kitchen Knife and Foldable Cutting Board Set: Children's Cooking Knives in 3 Sizes & Colors/Firm Grip, Serrated Edges, BPA-Free Kids' Knives/Safe Lettuce and Salad Knives

With Gratitude ...

First and foremost, I am grateful to my incredible husband David Bernstein whose love and support has been unwavering. His inspiration through his writing encouraged this publication.

I am blessed with an amazing supportive family: children Russell (Rachel), Jillian (Brooks), Chad (Marisa) and Jake (Nina) and sister Robin, who have all delighted in the meals I've prepared for them over the years and have provided me with valuable feedback.

Tina Moll — who has been helpful in cookbook structure, graphics and design.

Ann Jacobs, Bernadette Homan and Marianne Fisher, the marketing team at Arden Courts who are key supporters and friends who inspired me to publish this special *Power of 5 Test Kitchen Cookbook — Caregiver Edition*.

My dear friend Rochelle "Shelly" Brudny who provided her talent during the filming of the video counterpart to this cookbook.

My ChavaReads and Mahjong girlfriends who have been a constant encouragement and support during this adventure!

I am so grateful and appreciative to you all and to those I did not mention by name, you know who you are.

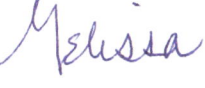

EMAIL MELISSA
Melissa@Powerof5TestKitchen.com

SUBSCRIBE
To receive delicious, healthy recipes directly in your inbox, sign up for Power of 5 Test Kitchen emails!
www.Powerof5TestKitchen.com

VISIT ON SOCIAL MEDIA
@Powerof5TestKitchen   @Powerof5TestKitchen

@DrDavidBernstein   Pinterest.com/DBernsteinMD

www.ingramcontent.com/pod-product-compliance
Lightning Source LLC
Chambersburg PA
CBHW042032150426
43200CB00002B/25